12 KEY HABITS TO THRIVE

JONATHAN ROCHE

Printed in the United States of America

Library of Congress Cataloging-in-Publication Data

ISBN: 9798818678795

I dedicate this book to my best friend and amazing wife, Karen, and my three remarkable children, Alex, Ben, and Adeline. You are my why, and I'm so blessed and grateful for the life we have together. Your love and support are gifts that allow me to pour myself into serving and positively impacting as many lives as humanly possible.

Thanks for making my life a joy and for being the reason I view myself as the luckiest person in the world!

CONTENTS

INTRODUCTION

With the Right Tools, You Can Thrive!

In the dictionary, the verb thrive is defined as "to prosper, be fortunate, or successful" and "to grow or develop vigorously." I believe that every person has the potential to thrive! No matter what your end goal, whether to reach your ideal weight, to receive a promotion at work, or to learn a new skill, like playing the piano, I believe that, if you have the right tools and put the work in, you can achieve those goals.

I have been blessed to be a Peak Performance Coach for over twenty years. I guide my clients in identifying, working toward, and attaining their goals. Through my work, I have learned that, when people do not meet their goals, when they think they have "failed," it is not because there is something wrong with them, it is because they do not have the right tools, specifically mental tools. So, you haven't struggled with your weight because you are lazy, lack willpower, or have bad genes. You haven't missed the mark on your career goals because you don't work hard enough, or because you aren't smart enough. The only differ-ence between people who are thriving and people who are struggling is a lack of mental tools to feel successful and achieve their goals. The mental tools I am talking about help you manage your thoughts, especially those thoughts that run through your mind that can lift you up or drag you down. Once you learn to have more control over the way you think, then you will feel free, and be able to hunt down your true potential and best self. And in doing so, you will begin to thrive and do it in a sustainable way

"Maybe the journey isn't so much about becoming anything. Maybe it's about un-becoming everything that isn't really you, so you can be who you were meant to be in the first place." —— Paulo Coelho

YOU DON'T NEED TO *CHANGE*—YOU JUST DESERVE TO *REVEAL.*

The high-energy, healthy, athletic, powerful, resourceful, bril-liant, and best version of yourself is inside of you and has been in there all along. You don't need to *change*, you simply deserve to *reveal* that version of you. She or he has been hidden until now due to you not having the awareness, tools, and strategies to control the voice in your mind. I am blessed and excited to be your guide as you take on your negative voice and reveal your best self!

As I will explain in this book, we all have both a negative voice and a positive voice in our heads. Our negative voice is our biggest critic and guides us in focusing on what is wrong (with us, with our body, with our spouse, with our job, etc.) and our positive voice is our biggest fan and guides us in focusing on what is right (with us, with our body, with our spouse, with our job, etc.). The key goal of this book is to guide you in controlling which voice is at the podium of your mind and then using that as rocket fuel to thrive.

Follow my lead, and let's begin the process of closing the gap between who you are and who you have the potential to be. I call this the "potential gap." True happiness and fulfillment are attained when you are "in the gap"—taking action; progressing toward your best self; making progress on your weight loss, health, and overall goals.

In this book, I'm going to guide you through winning the mental game and give you all the tools you need to thrive, both personally and professionally. Yes, you can hit your goal weight and stay there! Yes, you can crank up your energy and vibe and feel amazing! Yes, you can achieve your goals! But most important, you can gift yourself the best version of you. My goal is for this book to be one of the best and most impactful books you have read in your life. That is a lofty goal, but I think it's achievable, so lets do this!

Chapter One

THE REASON I WANT YOU TO THRIVE

Dory kept thinking her perpetual exhaustion was a product of her stressful life and her rapid pace. As a single mother of four, with kids ages 10, 12, 15, and 22, and juggling multiple jobs, she would end most days lying on the couch, exhausted.

But this exhaustion was different. It appeared that something was definitely wrong, so she finally went to the doctor. The doctor confirmed she was probably just run-down, but he ran some tests just to be sure. One of the tests included taking a look at her lungs, as the cough Dory had was getting worse and worse.

Then the dreaded call from the doctor came. The CT scan of her lungs came back with some alarming marks, and the doctor needed to see her right away. Over the next couple of days, more tests revealed scary and sad news: Dory was diagnosed with lung cancer, and it had been detected late. The news seemed like it could not get any worse, and then the doctor delivered the news that shook Dory to her core: she was given six months to live. She was only 47 years old.

About one year after being diagnosed and being given six months to live, Dory wrote the following letter to her children:

Sunday Jan 29, 1989

My dear dear Children,

I love you all so very much. I wanted to say how lucky I am to have each of you. You have been such wonderful children and given me so much joy in my life.

Please remember, you are never alone in this life — your dear friend and loving Father — God — is always there for you, and you will always have each other. Stay close all your lives — be best friends. Each of you is special and has so much to give to the world and to each other. Be happy, live life with confidence, love, peace and hope.

I'd hoped I'd be around a few more years — I wanted to see you all grow on and maybe bounce a grand child on my knee but it *appears that's not to be. So remember always — I'll have the next best thing — I'll be looking down from Heaven and see you all live such fine, loving, good and happy lives. You can always talk to me, still, as we always have. I'll always be listening and caring and loving you.*

Thank you for being my children and always being so wonderful to me. You made my life a joy.

Love,

Mom

On January 29, 1985, exactly 365 days after writing that letter, Dory Roche passed away. My beautiful mom was only 49 (she would have turned 50 four months later), and I was only 12.

My mom never met any of her eventual eleven grandchildren (including my three children, who are pictured here in October of 2021—Alexander is now 14, Benjamin is 12, and Adeline is 6).

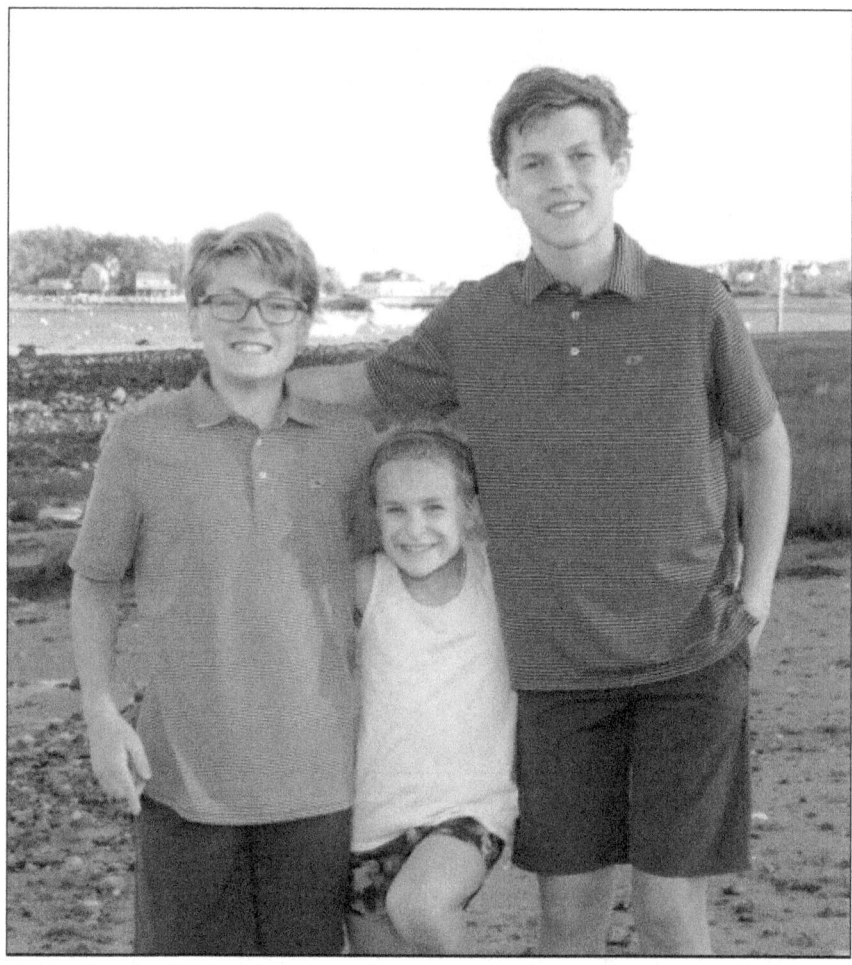

She had been a smoker and had always been trying to lose weight. But she never found the tools to get healthy and thrive, and she didn't have a chance to hit the re-start button on her health. You do! This is my motivation for providing tools for people to thrive. I not only want you to be around for as long as you can, but I also want the years that you are alive to be filled with growth and development. I want you to thrive!

Another part of my "why" is also personal. I have experienced my own transformation mentally, physically, and professionally. I will write more about my own experience in a later chapter, but in short, I was not always fit. I had been active in college, but when I started working full time at a finance job and was sitting at a desk for long hours each day, I started to put on weight. Before I knew it, I was 44 pounds overweight.

When I decided to focus on my health and to start to identify goals that would help me to thrive, I had to go through the same process that you are about to begin. I had to work on my mental game and start to incorporate all of the habits in this book into my daily life. I wrote this book because I lived it and still live it today!

I get it! I get the potential challenges and setbacks, but I also know firsthand the amazing way it feels when you are thriving —working toward your goals and achieving desired results. I am excited to share the tools and habits that have helped me to thrive because I truly believe everyone deserves to reveal their best self.

Chapter Two

THE IMPORTANCE OF HEALTH

I will talk a lot about health in this book, because you cannot thrive if you are not in good health. I am not saying that when you start to work toward thriving that you must be at your goal weight and with no health issues. But I am saying that part of thriving is *working toward* having good health. People who thrive are working toward a healthy weight and, eventually, achieving it and maintaining it. People who have health issues that are out of their control are working toward managing them and working with what they have to make opportunities to thrive in their lives.

REVERSE ENGINEER YOUR HEALTHY AND FUN LIFE

One of the best ways to create the healthy and fun life you want and deserve later in life (and now) is to follow the advice of the brilliant Stephen R. Covey (from his book *The 7 Habits of Highly Effective People*) and begin with the end in mind.

Please put your seatbelt on prior to reading this chapter, as it's about to get bumpy (not because I want to shock you, but because I want to save you and your family from disaster).

Here goes: There are essentially four ultimate *health-related* destinations in your life:

1. You die early from cancer or some other disease not tied directly to lifestyle.
2. You die early from heart disease, complications from diabetes, or from some other lifestyle disease that could have been avoided by making your health a top priority earlier in your life.
3. You live a long life but are stuck managing heart disease, high blood pressure, type 2 diabetes, etc., and feel terrible, have low-energy, and feel regret that could have been avoided by making your health a top priority earlier in life.
4. You live a long life, have taken care of your health, and are able to live independently at home and work full time (if you love your job) into your 80s or 90s. You move around with ease, go on hikes and long walks, and you are a source of positive energy and optimism for your family and friends. You are a glowing example of health and vitality, and you inspire others to say, "I want to be like her or him later in life!"

Now I want you to be candid with yourself. Up until right now, which ultimate destination have you chosen for yourself by the way you live each day?

Yes, I said "which have you *chosen*." I realize this is tough, and your negative voice is probably crying foul and trying to make me out as the bad guy. But this candid message has the potential to alter your life and your family, and even the ultimate destination of your children as adults.

My mom's best friend was Suzy (name changed to protect her identity, but her story is shared with permission). She has looked after me since my mom passed away when I was 12, and she is like my second mom. My kids call her Nana, and we are blessed to have her in our lives.

Suzy is now 85. She lived in the same home she raised her six children in until she was 83 and now lives alone in a townhouse. She exercises seven mornings per week (walking five miles), and she worked full time until she was 83. Suzy feels drastically younger than her age. She started exercising in her 30s after being surprised and disappointed with not being able to keep up with a friend who had invited Suzy to exercise with her. That was her turning point, and 55 years later, she is still going.

When I posted a "Happy 84th Birthday" message to Suzy on my Facebook page (along with a picture of her), a person asked her:

> "How do you look sooooo young? Do you have joint pain which needs mental-overcoming in order to stay active? If not, do you use anything to keep joints pain-free? Or do you just ignore pain and keep moving? Please share any tips."

Here is Suzy's reponse:

> "Actually, I am lucky enough to not have any pain anywhere right now. I truly believe that's because I have stayed active. Jonathan knows the drill. Follow his lead."

In contrast, Suzy's husband (I'll call him Joe) never made his health a top priority. He was never overweight, but he didn't exercise or watch what he ate. He just did his thing, and over time, it caught up with him. Joe spent his final two years living in a nursing home and needing a walker to get around. He needed 24-hour care, and my kids and I would go to visit Grandpa Joe and feel sad and shocked by how different his life was compared to Suzy's. Suzy went and visited him every day, and one of the saddest things is that a lot of his issues could have been avoided if Joe had made his health a top priority.

Beyond the sad state of his health and what that did to hinder quality time with his wife and family (they have six kids and eight grandkids), their life savings was running out fast, because the nursing home Joe lived in was $12,400 per month. *Per month*!

One day, during the first few months of Joe being at the nursing home, Suzy went to visit him. The nurses at the front desk told Suzy, "We think your dad is our nicest resident!" Suzy had taken such good care of herself that some at the nursing home thought Joe was her father!

In May of 2018, Suzy called me to let me know that doctors thought Joe only had a few days to live. I went to the nursing home to see him. Joe and I had a pleasant conversation about my three kids, and then he thanked me for always looking out for Suzy. When I went to say my final goodbye to Joe and give him a hug, he pulled me in close. We were eye to eye, and he said, "Jonathan, do it differently than I did it. Take care of yourself and your health so that you don't end up like me." Then he smiled and said it again, "Do it differently, and take care of yourself, Jonathan!" He smiled, and I smiled, and I said my final goodbye. Joe passed away a few days later.

Who do you want to be when you are in your 80s? Suzy or Joe? Beyond using this story to light a fire within you, my hope is that you see how important it is, not only to take care of your health so that you feel good and have a high quality of life as you age, but also to see how your health can affect those around you. If you keep in mind what you want your later years to look and feel like for you and your loved ones, my hope is that it is one more motivator to make your health a top priority. Sharing this story is a way for me to honor Joe and to pass on his final words of wisdom to me:

"Do it differently and take care of yourself!"

Harness the power of beginning with the end in mind. Choose to focus on your health, as it's one of the greatest gifts you will ever give yourself, and it is key to thriving in all areas of your life.

Chapter Three

HIT THE RE-START BUTTON

"It is never too late to be what you might have been." — George Eliot

Your negative voice has maybe fooled you into believing it's too late to drop the weight, get fit, run the 10K, do the triathlon, make the career change, chase your dreams, etc., but the powerful quote from George Eliot above is the truth. It's never too late!

My mom's best friend, Suzy, who I wrote about earlier and who I use as my role model of someone who set herself up to be healthy and active later in life, didn't start running until she was in her 50s! She ran for 30 years and just recently switched to walking. She still participates in, and finishes, 5Ks. In fact, she says she has won every 5K she has entered since turning 70, usually because she is the only person in her age group!

Here is another powerful example of living out George Eliot's quote: This is an email I received in 2016:

Email Title: I want you to coach me 1-on-1

"Hi, Jonathan,

My name is Jen, and I'm writing because I want to hire you as my coach. I saw your offer to do 20 weeks of phone coaching, but I wanted to check with you prior to grabbing a spot. You see, I have terminal brain cancer, but I am choosing to chase down my dreams anyway. One of my big dreams is to run a marathon. I was signed up for one and training when I was diagnosed, and when the day of the marathon came, I was devastated. But then I got over my pity party and decided I would train for next year. Will you coach me? I am planning on doing the marathon next year, and I know I can do it with you as my personal coach. Let me know."

I was blessed to coach Jen, and she did complete her marathon. Jen decided she would not let her circumstances define her or hinder her. She and Suzy are glowing examples of hitting the re-start button!

Another example of someone who hit the re-start button is my father. My dad had times in his life when he was thriving. He was a running back on the Boston College Division 1 football team and then had a successful career as he began to build his family. But that successful career became hectic, and the stresses of his life led to him carrying around an extra 50–75 pounds and all the health issues that come with the excess weight. He also struggled with alcoholism for years but hit the re-start button at the end of his life. He went to AA and remained sober for his six final years.

While at AA, he used his experiences to help others on their own journey. My father passed away in 1995 at the age of 62 (I was 23). His wake was packed with people he had served. Many came through the line at his wake, sharing story after story of how my dad had helped them. It was a powerful experience to hear the positive impact he had made on these people and the world. He was able to accomplish this because he wasn't afraid to re-start.

BE A CYCLE-BREAKER

One of the ways I honor my parents is to be a cycle-breaker. I consciously chose to focus on and work on my health, well-being and mindset so that I can live longer and be healthier than the previous generation. How about you? Maybe your parents are still around but struggling with their weight, health and mindset. Or maybe they have passed after struggling with their weight, health and mindset. Either way, the greatest way to honor your parents is to be a cycle-breaker.

Your negative voice might hear that and say, "That sounds rude or like you are being disrespectful to your parents," but it's the opposite. You are actually honoring them by breaking the cycle, since you are about to have the tools that they didn't have to drop weight for good, to get healthy, and to thrive. My parents were great people, but they didn't have the tools like the 12 Key Habits to Thrive. Maybe your parents didn't have the tools or don't have the tools. But now you do (everything you need is in this book), and now is your chance to break the cycle of an unhealthy lifestyle, so that your kids and future generations don't have to struggle with their weight, health or mindset. You can be one of the first in your family to start a new way of life in which you can thrive.

Here is some scary, but highly-motivating, research from the American Academy of Childhood Psychiatry:

- A child with one obese parent (30 or more pounds overweight) has a 50% likelihood of becoming an obese adult.
- A child with two obese parents (30 or more pounds overweight) has an 80% likelihood of becoming an obese adult.

We work so hard to teach our children how to thrive and to pass on positive habits (treating people right, working hard, being of service to others, etc.). But what most people don't realize is that we also pass on our lifestyles. Let's honor our parents by breaking the cycle, and in doing so, gift our kids with the type of healthy lifestyle and mindset that they deserve to thrive in life!

YOUR PAST IS NOT YOUR FUTURE

As you focus on working through the 12 Habits and beginning to thrive, your negative voice will try to convince you that this attempt isn't going to work. It will try to come up with evidence of past failures and frustrations that will make you question whether you can succeed this time. I want you to remember this:

YOUR PAST IS NOT YOUR FUTURE!

Just because you've made other attempts to reach your goals that didn't work out, doesn't mean this attempt can't be different. Too many people label themselves based on their past, particularly when it comes to weight loss, and you deserve better. There's nothing you can do about decisions you've already made, so hammering yourself about weight you've gained, workouts you've missed, or food you ate, only takes you in the wrong direction. In fact, when you spend time (*any* time) thinking about yesterday's missteps, you're using energy you could be putting into *winning today and thriving*.

I have an important request. Don't let yesterday's slipups rob you of today's and tomorrow's victories! Give yourself permission to focus on what you can do today and not what you have done in the past. Once you do that, you free yourself to put 100% of your energy into winning today, by focusing on things you can do, *starting immediately*. And it's simple: You can drink water, eat every two to three hours, fit in your workout, work on your mental game, and be grateful for what you have. And as we will talk about later, gratitude goes a long way toward building healthy habits and thriving!

In order to get a realistic picture of what you have been focusing on each day, please complete the following exercise.

Give percentages of the amount of time during an average day that you spend focusing on each of these:

The Past: Looking back at yesterday (being lectured by your negative voice about missed workouts, bad nutritional choices, weight you have put back on, missed work deadlines, times when presentations did not go as well as you had hoped, etc.)

The Present: Looking at today (how much water you have had, when you are working out, the work you accomplished for the day, how you are incorporating the 12 Habits to Thrive into your life, etc.)

The Future: Looking forward (how you are going to lose 30 pounds by the end of the year, how you can stay consistent with your goals for the entire month, etc.)

Honestly rate each of these, and then spend two minutes looking at your answers and thinking about them.

What would happen to your fitness, weight loss, and other goals if you put 100% of your energy into today? What would this do for your mental peace of mind? What would this do as far as reducing your stress?

When (not *if*) you put 100% of your energy into making today remarkable and nailing your healthy habits, amazing things will happen, and your rocket will leave the pad! Embrace the fact that today is a new day, and you can't do anything to change yesterday—but you *can* put all your effort into winning today.

MAKE TODAY JANUARY 1

Many people put a big emphasis on starting a new fitness and weight-loss plan or new personal development program on January 1. While it's always great to have goals with specific timelines, this particular one has become too powerful and makes people discouraged when they are not successful. It also can lead to thinking that, if you didn't stick to your plan during the first weeks of the new year, you should just give up.

Research shows that 80% of people bail on their New Year's resolutions by the end of week two, and 98% bail by the end of week four! Why do we think we "blew it" because we didn't achieve our grand plan of losing X amount of weight or quitting smoking by the end of January? Don't take score too soon! You can begin again any day of the year. Why wait until January 1 to start doing amazing things with your energy and health?

If you started the year with solid intentions, but never got going, or forgot about them a few weeks in, then today is a great day to begin again. Any day can be the start of something amazing, so make today your January 1. Forget about however many weeks or months have passed this year—that's now water under the bridge.

Remember, focusing on yesterday is focusing on something you can't change and is only going to drag you in the wrong direction. Jump in and make today your January 1. Then get excited to crush it over the remaining weeks of the year!

How about you? What big dreams and goals have you had that you have shelved because you thought it was too late? Now is the time to pull them out and give them a go. Everything you need to meet your goals and to thrive is in this book—*every-thing*—and you have the option, right now, to hit the re-start button.

Think about it: You can completely reinvent yourself (mentally, physically, spiritually, and emotionally) and inspire those around you to do the same.

Don't put off revealing the high-energy and healthy version of yourself that lies within. Most people never reach their potential and, instead, just accept going with the flow. They keep putting off their dreams and goals until, one day later in life, they start asking themselves hard questions like "What could I have done, or who could I have become, if I'd just gone for it?" Don't let that be you. Every one of us has unique greatness in us that is ready to be unlocked. Don't be afraid to re-start and get going.

Chapter Four

THE 12 KEY HABITS TO THRIVE

I want you to look at your reinvention, and the process of permanently achieving your goals, like building a house. The key to an amazing house is to make sure that you build a foundation that is so strong it can handle anything.

The 12 Key Habits to Thrive will form the rock-solid foundation of the new you. Once you understand these 12 Key Habits, then apply them and live them, you will be equipped to achieve the goals you set. The habits are mainly focused on your mindset and on health. Since a great number of people have a goal of reaching their ideal weight, several of the health habits contain examples that are centered around weight loss.

No matter what your goal, however, the habits are implemented in a similar fashion. The habits are about living a lifestyle that will allow you to set and reach goals, thus allowing you to thrive. Each habit will be discussed in its own chapter but for now, here is a list of the 12 Key Habits to Thrive.

1. **Nail Your Voice Choice**
2. **Focus on Your Energy**
3. **Control Your Stress**
4. **Have an Attitude of Gratitude**
5. **Upgrade Your Team and Embrace Being a Leader**
6. **Embrace Being Your Own Effort-Based Head Coach**
7. **Exercise and Be a Random Acts of Fitness Machine**
8. **Form Your Lifestyle/Career Around Your Wellness**
9. **Commit to the 7-Day Week**
10. **Plan for Success**
11. **Set Insanely Big Goals**
12. **Use Positive Content to Win the Mental Game**

The above habits are your foundation to begin to thrive. If you follow these, you will be set up to achieve your goals. As you began to work with these habits, I want to remind you that there is no reason to rush through them. In fact, if you take your time and really incorporate the habits into your life, they will be more sustainable. When it comes to thriving and meeting your goals, you really have two options:

YOU CAN HURRY UP AND FAIL, OR YOU CAN TAKE YOUR TIME AND WIN!

What I mean by "hurry up and fail" is to make major changes to your habits that are unsustainable. As I mentioned before, each

January, people get all fired up to take action on their New Year's resolutions. They do long workouts and/or try some crazy diet. They practice a new skill for hours and hours until they begin to lose their motivation. They are able to keep at it for two to four weeks, and then they drop off. They have "hurried up and failed."

The second option is the one I'm coaching and guiding you on in this book. It's also the option I've been coaching and guiding others on for over 20 years. I call it "take your time and win." You don't need to rush into the 12 Habits. These habits are sustainable, and you should be able to do them for the rest of your life. Yes, you would like to get to your goal weight as soon as possible or get that raise tomorrow. But more important than how quickly you get there, is the fact that, by using the 12 Key Habits, you are going to *stay* there.

Chapter Five

KEY HABIT #1: NAIL YOUR VOICE CHOICE

As I mentioned earlier, we all have two voices in our heads—a negative voice and a positive voice.

Your negative voice guides you to focus on what is wrong with everything, like your job, your house, your partner, your kids, your body, etc. It is that inner critic that we all have that talks down to us. It points out our missteps and keeps us from staying on track. When you listen to your negative voice, you get dragged down, mentally, physically and emotionally.

Your positive voice, on the other hand, guides you to focus on what is right with the world, with your house, with your job, with your partner, with your kids, and with you. Your positive voice is your biggest fan and will guide you in taking action on habits that fuel your energy, health, vitality, productivity, optimism, gratitude, and happiness. It helps us stay on track and to reframe setbacks, not as failure, but as a step on our journey. *Webster's Dictionary* defines "hope" as "the feeling that what is wanted can be had or that events will turn out for the best." This is the essence of your positive voice.

Now, imagine that there is a podium in your mind. At any given moment, you get to choose who stands at the podium and speaks. This is your voice choice. Who will you allow to speak, and therefore, who will you choose to listen to?

Your response to everything is a product of your voice choice. This is a simple statement, but it's spot on and it's powerful. Every action you take, everything you do, how you interact with your partner, kids, friends, coworkers, etc., is a product of whether you choose to allow your negative voice or your positive voice to speak at the podium of your mind. That decision (that you make every day and numerous times per day) is the difference between a mediocre life and a life in which you thrive.

In addition to the way we treat ourselves, the way we treat others is also a product of our voice choice. If our positive voice is at the podium, we are generally positive, supportive, patient, empathic, and loving. But when our negative voice is at the podium, we are generally impatient, stressed, and unsupportive. Also, our ability to treat everyone the same (with dignity and respect) decreases when our negative voice is at the podium. My dad believed that everyone should receive good and positive energy from others. Here is a quote from him that is easy to act on when our positive voice is at the podium but difficult when our negative voice is at the podium:

"Everyone gets the good stuff! Treat the garbage man the same way you treat a CEO. Giving respect is free and easy!" — Don Roche, Sr.

Our voice choice also impacts our accomplishments and our ability to take action. There are two types of people in the world: Talkers and Doers. Talkers sit around and talk about what they hope to do and what they plan to do.

Doers take action. They are in the game, attempting to improve themselves, following through on their commitments, completing tasks, and chasing down their goals and dreams.

Guess which inner voice is at the podium in each of these two groups? Yes, you guessed it. Talkers are guided by their negative voice. Doers are guided by their positive voice!

Now you can see how important and impactful your voice choice is.

You must win the mental game before you can position yourself to meet your goals and thrive. Mindset always comes before action when it comes to lasting transformation. So let's talk about how you can learn to nail your voice choice!

"If you give a fool a stage, he or she will perform." — Unknown

Your negative voice will perform (talk down to you) all day long if you give her or him the stage. The key is to remove your negative voice from the podium and intentionally and consistently invite your positive voice to the podium. Once this is accomplished, it's game over as far as you revealing your best self.

Nailing your voice choice has two phases:

1. Control your inner dialogue.
2. Empower your positive voice.

CONTROL YOUR INNER DIALOGUE

There are four phases of controlling your inner dialogue:

Phase #1: Acceptance

Phase #2: Identification

Phase #3: Awareness

Phase #4: Implementing Voice Choice

PHASE #1: ACCEPTANCE

Some people don't realize that they have a negative voice. They have never identified or thought much about that inner critic that talks down to them. Some people even believe they don't have a negative voice at all. But what they don't realize is that everyone has a voice in their head that can get in the way of their progress and goals.

In fact, I believe that every person on this planet (including professional athletes, Olympic athletes, music superstars, and CEOs of major companies) has a negative voice. The reason they are still able to thrive at a high level is that they have learned and implemented tools and strategies to control that voice.

Here is a quote from country music superstar Tim McGraw, from his biography *Grit & Grace*:

> "Back in this period, I didn't have strategies for living with this duality. I wasn't comfortable sitting back, watching and waiting in stillness. In hindsight, I think it's because if things got quiet, I'd hear the old ghosts that tend to follow at my heels like shadows. The ones that say, *You're just a small-town country singer on a lucky streak—what do you know about success?*" — *Tim McGraw*

Here is another quote about one of the greatest Ironman triathletes in history, Mark Allen, regarding his battle with his negative voice prior to winning his first of six Ironman World Championships:

> "Mark heard a voice in his head at the most critical moments of the race. The same confidence-crushing script played over and over: *I can't do it! This guy's too strong! I'm going to lose again!* Despite his talent, his love of swimming, his willingness to work hard, and a burning desire to win, Mark carried a deep sense of self-doubt into his racing that made him weak in the moments when he most needed to be strong. Any endurance athlete can fall prey to a voice of negativity and self-pity in crisis moments, but in Mark that mutinous inner voice had a special personal significance. It *hated* him." — from *Ironwar* by Matt Fitzgerald

As you can see, even very successful people have a negative voice. The difference is that they are aware of it and have learned to control it. Accepting that you have a negative voice is a key first step in your journey to controlling your inner dialogue.

PHASE #2: IDENTIFICATION

Now that we know that everyone has a negative voice, it is important to know the different ways in which your negative voice can present itself. Some of these may seem obvious, like the inner critic that talks down to you. Some, however, may be more of a surprise. Some versions can actually seem supportive and kind, but if what they are saying at the podium of your mind is getting in the way of you meeting your goals and thriving, that is a negative voice.

I have identified three versions of your negative voice. As you read these descriptions, think about which version(s) you have:

1. The Bully: This version says rude things like "What is wrong with you?" or guides you in using words like "fat" to describe yourself. This is the worst version of the negative voice, because it talks down to you and makes you feel terrible about yourself. That is why I named it "Bully." By the way, the word fat is degrading and should *never be used* while speaking, or within your own thoughts. You deserve better. So, if you have used that word, let's put an end to that starting today.

2. The Distractor: This version distracts you from taking action on the key habits that lead to you thriving. An

example is saying something like "You have too much going on at work, so you better skip your morning workout, so you can get to the office" or "The kids' schedules are crazy today, so you should work on that report later." The Distractor is not obviously negative, like the Bully, but it's just as destructive as far as holding you back from your goals and from thriving.

3. The Buddy: This version comes across like a friend who is looking out for you, so I named it The Buddy. It only shows up in two situations: When you are cranking along, dropping weight and/or making other progress, or if you are in a state of turmoil (someone in your family is sick, during a health pandemic, etc.).

Here are some examples of The Buddy in action:

"You're dropping 1.5 pounds per week, so it's not a big deal to have an extra dessert."

"Your mom is sick, so you should blow off your health and put 100% of your focus into her."

"We are in the middle of a health pandemic, so let's shelve our career goals until we get through it. There is no sense in working hard now."

Do any of these versions of negative voice sound familiar? Once you are able to identify the different kinds of negative voice you may have, you will be better able to control your inner dialogue.

PHASE #3: AWARENESS

It's important to be aware of how big an opportunity you have as far as shifting your inner dialogue. Please note that I use the word "opportunity," instead of "problem," as we work through how loud your negative voice is and how often it takes over your podium. Most people's scarcest commodity is time. It seems like we are all in a constant state of not having enough time. By quantifying how much time you spend listening to, or in discussions with, your negative voice, you will see how big an opportunity you have to take back hours per day, which you can then invest in meeting your goals and thriving.

I created the below Inner Dialogue (ID) Score, to help quantify this time spent engaging with your negative voice.

TAKE YOUR INNER DIALOGUE (ID) SCORE

Step 1: Add up the total amount of time you spend per day dealing with each version of your negative voice. Here is a hint: For nine out of ten people, it is *hours* per day—not minutes.

Example: 2 hours per day.

Step 2: Take your number from Step #1 and multiply it by 365. The answer will be the number of hours per *year* you spend in discussions with, or fending off, your negative voice.

Example: 2 hours X 365 days = 730 hours per year

· · ·

Step 3: Come up with the average number of hours you are awake per day by subtracting the number of hours you sleep per night from 24.

Example: I sleep 7 hours per night, so 24 – 7 = 17 hours.

Step 4: Divide your answer from Step #2 (hours per year) by your answer from Step #3 (the amount of time you are awake per day) to come up with the total days per year you are spending in dialogue or fending off your negative voice.

Example: 730 hours per year divided by 17 hours of average awake time per day = 43 days per year.

This number is your starting Inner Dialogue (ID) Score. I suggest you retake your score every 30 days and focus on lowering your score over time!

The higher your ID Score, the more excited you should be! Why? Because you have achieved amazing things with a less than 12-month year. During the hours you are dealing with your negative voice, you are not able to take action on your goals. Therefore, taking this time back is a huge opportunity!

For instance, using the numbers from the above example: You have only had 10.5- month years (since 43 days out of the year have been spent with your negative voice), so think of how much you are going to be able to crank up your results as you gain back the time.

Now you can identify your negative voice in its different forms, and you are aware of how much time you spend engaging with your negative voice. You also have a way to quantify the progress you make each month by taking your updated ID Score. So now let's learn some tools and strategies to help you with your voice choice.

PHASE #4: IMPLEMENTING VOICE CHOICE

Implementing voice choice includes fending off your negative voice, as well as empowering your positive voice. Once you have mastered these two things, you will know how to invite your positive voice to the podium so that it can cheer you on to thrive.

Here are some tips for fending off each of the three versions of your negative voice:

THE BULLY:

1. Refuse to engage in a discussion. Just like with real bullies, if you don't respond to their nonsense, they will give up on bothering you.
2. Come up with a quick comeback statement like "Go away!" or "Not today!" or "You're invisible to me!"
3. When being lectured by your Bully voice about not being perfect, I suggest saying, "Who cares?" It doesn't mean that you don't care about *results*. It just means "Who cares?" if you didn't nail every *detail*—you are human.

THE DISTRACTOR:

1. Have a "7-day week" mindset (Key Habit #9, which I go over later in the book). Commit to being healthy and focused seven days per week. Many people get off track, because they are only fully committed on weekdays or, when it comes to health, especially weight loss, consistently allow themselves "cheat days." The noncommitted time then cancels out all of their hard work from their committed time. By having a 7-day week mindset, you have a plan in place to ignore The Distractor and stay focused and committed.

2. Refuse to use the "I don't have time" excuse. If you are spending time on social media or watching TV (which many of us do), you do have time. By refusing to use this excuse, when The Distractor tries to talk you out of a workout, out of completing a work project, or out of completing the Win Tomorrow Checklist (another tool you will learn about later in the book), you can simply say, "I have the time and I'm doing it!"

THE BUDDY:

1. Keep your goals in mind by writing them down and rereading them each morning and night. Then, when The Buddy shows up, you can say things to yourself like, "I deserve to feel remarkable more than I deserve an extra dessert!" or "The reason I feel so amazing is because I don't skip workouts just, because I'm

rocking it!" Reminding yourself twice daily about what you are working toward, and how you feel when you stay with your plan to achieve your goals, will help you stay committed.

2. When you are in a crisis or in the middle of a health pandemic, remind yourself that you feel good and get positive energy from working toward your goals. Say things to yourself like, "I need to be as positive and energized as possible to handle this additional stress, so I am going to stick to my plan."

EMPOWER YOUR POSITIVE VOICE

The best way to empower your positive voice is to practice giving it attention. Intentionally ask, and be aware of, what your positive voice would say in any situation. Really ask yourself, "What does my positive voice think?"

It's easy to look at that question and be fooled by its simplicity. But asking yourself what your positive voice thinks on a frequent basis can be life-altering. It completely shifts your focus.

Remember, these skills take practice. Most people have spent years with their negative voice at the podium of their minds. It will take some time to empower your positive voice to start to take over.

One way to help ensure success is to be intentional each morning about listening to your positive voice. Before your feet hit the floor, say to yourself, "I'm going to listen to my positive voice today!" Then do periodic check-ins throughout the day. Ideally, these check-ins should happen every two or three hours. Set up reminders on your phone or watch! This can be as simple as "Nail your voice choice" or "Who is at the Podium?" reminders.

For 99% of people, not choosing their positive voice each morning means they, by default (subconsciously), choose their negative voice. Your ability to control your inner dialogue (fending off your negative voice, while empowering your positive voice) is pivotal to meeting your goals and reaching your potential. The way you speak to yourself will dictate the quality of your life. Of all the things you can focus on when it comes to working toward your goals and thriving, controlling your inner dialogue should be priority number one.

COMPARING YOUR THOUGHTS BASED ON YOUR VOICE CHOICE

> "When we change the way we look at things, the things we look at change." — Wayne Dyer

I created the below chart so that you can see a side-by-side comparison of how different your life and experiences are when your positive voice is at the podium compared to your negative voice. If you notice a reaction when you read about a particular situation on the chart, that may be a clue as to where you can find your negative voice. This information will help you become more aware of where your negative voice comes out in its various forms.

As you will see in this chart, your negative voice leads to negativity on your journey, and your positive voice leads to positivity and the ability to thrive. When you work to put your positive voice at the podium of your mind, you set yourself up to thrive.

Here is a quote that speaks to the shift that is about to happen for you:

> "Your biggest challenge isn't someone else; it's the ache in your lungs, the burning in your legs, and the voice inside you that yells 'can't,' but you don't listen. You push harder. And then you hear the voice whisper 'can.' And you discover that the person you thought you were is no match for the one you really are." — Unknown

Comparing your Thoughts based on your Voice Choice		
Situation	**Negative Voice**	**Positive Voice**
Focus (in general):	What is wrong Non-controllables Perfectionism All-or-nothing thinking	What is right Controllables Progress If I stumble, I get back on the horse
Focus (as far as how you are doing):	What you are doing wrong How far you are from your goal Lectures and shames you about what you are doing wrong	What you are doing right. How far you have come Cheers you on and loves how many things you are doing right
Approach to cheering you on:	Your loudest critic	Your biggest fan
Self-care approach:	Grind (learned exhaustion) Avoids nourishing of mind/body	Extreme self-care (pacing) Nourishes mind/body
Top priority:	Everyone else (you aren't on the list)	You and your own health
Response to requests on your time:	Likes to say yes to everything.	Is comfortable saying no
Self-coaching approach:	Results-based coach	Effort-based coach
Weigh-ins:	Judgment/shame Defines whether you have a good or bad day	One of many ways to measure success. It's just data
Standards and expectations:	None or low	Defined and high
Approach to leadership:	Avoids leadership	Embraces leadership
Labels:	Disempowering labels (Lazy and other rude terms, like the one that starts with F and ends with T)	Empowering labels (Powerful, smart, resilient, fun, athletic, caring, kind, funny, resourceful, etc.)
Approach to desired transformation:	Change: You need to change (guilt, shame & judgment)	Reveal: You deserve to reveal (Your best self is already in there and is ready to be revealed.)
Approach to planning:	Dislikes planning and prefers to wing it	Plans and systematizes to remove thinking time and maximize follow-through
Approach to others (family, coworkers, etc.)	Focus on what they are doing wrong	Focus on what they are doing right
Time perspective:	Wants instant gratification	Is comfortable with delayed gratification
Comparison to:	Everyone else	Your prior self
Response to other's success:	Jealous	Inspired
Typical Energy Level (from 0 to 5):	0 - 3	3 - 5
Typical Stress Level (from 0 to 5):	3 - 5	0 - 3
Typical Happiness (from 0 to 5):	0 - 3	3 - 5

ONE ADDITIONAL IMPORTANT POINT: YOU WILL NEVER PLEASE YOUR NEGATIVE VOICE.

Many people spend their entire lives trying to please their inner critic. But the sad fact is that whatever we do will never be enough to please our negative voice. There will never be enough weight dropped or success achieved, and the bar will continually be raised. Many people spend their entire lives set up to fail, trying to please their negative voice. Then, near the end of their journey on this Earth, they realize they were fooled. They spent their life with a negative copilot, and they were playing a game they could never win. But at that point it's too late.

But, luckily, that is not you. By giving me the blessing of being your guide through this book, you now know that you deserve to ditch your negative voice, empower your positive voice, and unleash the high-energy, positive, fit, healthy, and happy version of yourself who has been in there all along. You are now free to soar!

I want to end this chapter by reiterating something extremely important: The most important decision of your life happens every morning when you wake up: Which voice are you going to listen to—your negative voice or your positive voice?

Choose your positive voice and enjoy the journey!

Chapter Six

KEY HABIT #2: FOCUS ON YOUR ENERGY

When we set out to accomplish our goals, we can sometimes get overwhelmed by the enormity of the process. We can also spend too much time focusing on each small detail, which can make us feel like giving up before we start.

As I have coached people, I have found that, when they focus on their overall energy, rather than the details, they are more successful. The kind of energy I am talking about is more about how you are *feeling* rather than if you are moving through life at a rapid pace. Although, if you feel good, you typically can get more done each day.

Ensuring that your energy is positive and empowering sets you up to work toward your goals. Life is drastically easier when your energy level is high. Why? Because the little things don't bother you, and you give off a positive feeling and vibe that draws people to you. Put another way: You draw in positive people and things, and you also repel negative people.

One simple thing to do to begin focusing on your energy is to check in with yourself multiple times each day about what your current energy level is. A key way to do this is to ask yourself a simple, but powerful, question:

What is my energy level? (On a scale of 0 to 5: 0 = you are dragging and 5 = you are on fire.)

If you answer 4 or 5, then keep doing what you're doing. If you answer 3 or less, ask yourself the next logical question: "What can I do to crank up my energy?"

EARN YOUR LEVEL 5 ENERGY AND THEN GUARD IT

When your energy level is at 5, you feel amazing, and not surprisingly, your happiness level goes through the roof. You truly feel mentally, physically, and emotionally great, and you also feel fulfilled for doing the best you can. So how do you get there?

One way is to change your language. A lot of people focus on what they *have* to do when they are working toward their goals instead of what they *get* to do. This simple shift in language can lay the groundwork to change the lens through which you view doing the more challenging work toward your goals.

For example, instead of saying, "I *have* to work out today," say, "I *get* to work out today." Instead of saying, "I *have* to write this report for work," say, "I *get* to write this report." It is only human to feel overwhelmed at times, with all the things we have to get done, especially when we set big goals for ourselves. However, if you try to give it a more positive spin in your mind, it will help shift your entire attitude toward the hard stuff!

Another way you can increase your positive energy is to focus on putting your positive voice at the podium of your mind. As I discussed in the previous chapter, this move alone will help you win the mental game daily! It will allow you to focus on being healthy overall, eating the right foods, and getting in daily movement and exercise.

A final way to increase your positive energy is to consume positive content. Read motivational books and watch movies that inspire you. The more we expose ourselves to positive content, the more we absorb it, and the more likely it is to become a strong part of our mental game.

WHAT DO YOU SAY TO PEOPLE BEFORE YOU SPEAK?

"Your energy announces you to the room before you speak." — Unknown

It's key to realize that your energy and vibe announce you (in person, on Zoom, on a call, etc.) before you speak. Prior to reading this book and shifting your focus to cranking up your energy, what do you think you were saying to people before you spoke? Were you giving off positive energy and, therefore, drawing people toward you, or were you giving off negative energy and inadvertently pushing people away?

If you feel like you are not presenting yourself to others with the best energy, maybe you are living out what I call "learned exhaustion." Learned exhaustion is a state of perpetual exhaustion that has been your normal state for so long that you have learned to live with it and just *be* it. You have been so busy juggling so many things that you have gradually, over time, between not getting enough sleep and doing too much, shifted into a perpetual state of exhaustion. This is not good for your long-term health, and it's really bad for your energy, vibe, and happiness. Hopefully, you have already started to shift away from this state (at least in your head, which is the place to start) as you read through this book.

If you have been in a state of learned exhaustion, then I'm excited to be guiding you to the energized, positive, and healthy version of yourself that you deserve. We are focused on today and moving forward, so go all in on earning your level 5 energy!

YOU CAN'T GIVE AWAY WHAT YOU DON'T HAVE

Another reason to focus on cranking up your energy to level 5 is so that you can gift some of it to others when they need it. This is sort of like what they tell you on airplanes, that you need to put on your own oxygen mask before you can help others.

Most people *want* to help others, and it can make us feel really good to help others. But if we aren't taking care of ourselves and making sure *our* energy levels are high and positive, we won't have enough to give away. Or if we do give to others, it will leave us feeling drained and depleted.

After you have made focusing on your energy part of your life, you will consistently have your energy bucket filled up to level

5. Eventually, you will not only have your own energy bucket filled up to level 5, but you will have a second bucket filled as well! You can use that extra bucket when a family member, friend, coworker, stranger, etc., needs a lift or a helping hand. Yes, it takes considerable effort to get to level 5 and to, potentially, fill up a second bucket. But the effort is well worth it when you see the positive impact you have on others!

EARN YOUR AWESOME

When someone asks you how you are doing, what is your typical answer? If you are like most people, you probably say "fine" or "good" or possibly "great." Or, if you're having a tough day, maybe just "okay." When we answer with okay, fine, good, or even great, it is almost as if the person is not even registering your answer, because it isn't a pattern interrupt.

Your answer to the question "How are you?" usually correlates with your energy level. This is key to keep in mind, as you shift from focusing on the small steps of attaining your goals to focusing on your energy. Imagine you have earned your level 5 energy, and someone asks you how you are doing. You'd probably use words like "amazing," "fantastic," or even "awesome!" What type of response do you think you would receive from your answer? I can answer that for you. He or she would smile and get a lift from you, and about 25% of people would make a comment, like "I want to feel awesome too!" or "I love that answer!" or "What do you do to feel awesome?"

Below is a story that speaks to the power of focusing on your energy and the power of "earning your awesome."

In October of 2019, I arrived early at San Diego Airport to fly back to Boston. I had just been blessed to speak at a conference to 2,000 people, and one of the topics I covered was "Earn Your Awesome!" In fact, my team and I had given out "Earn Your Awesome!" bracelets at our booth.

As I share the rest of this story, I invite you to consider a few key things:

1. I train for life's biggest events, and I suggest you do as well. No, I don't mean you should start running. I use the word "train" as a reference to preparation. You can train for a big meeting, a presentation, a speaking engagement, or even for your family vacation (this way you are fully present for your vacation, rather than wasting one to two days at the start, as you come out of your over-worked fog). To train just means to elevate your commitment to follow through on the key areas of wellness (water, sleep, nutrients, exercise, and positive content). I was trained and ready to go for my speaking engagement, and that led to me feeling amazing and still at an energy level of 5 after the event (and as I headed to the airport).

2. I had made the key decision that morning (as I do every morning) to invite my positive voice to the podium and had done periodic check-ins throughout the day to make sure that continued. So, as I arrived at the airport, my positive voice was still in control of my thoughts and actions.

3. Not only was I at an energy level of 5, but I had a

second bucket of energy (that I had been filling over
many months and years) available to share with others.

Okay, back to the story. Since I was two hours early, I decided to
go have an early lunch. After finishing a chicken sandwich, my
negative voice tried to convince me to finish the french fries too.
I fought it off and, instead, asked for my check. I point this out
because, if I had stayed and finished the fries, the precise timing
of the encounters I'm about to share would not have happened.

While paying the bill, a Marine walked by, and my immediate
thought was "I'm going to pay for that guy's lunch." My negative voice tried to talk me out of it with things like, "You will
look strange," etc., but I fought off the voice. Instead, I paid my
bill, pulled $25 from my wallet, and walked over to the Marine.
Now, I will point out again that, if my negative voice had won
this battle, the timing would have been off, and I would have
missed out on two more powerful encounters that were about
to happen.

I walked up to the Marine, extended my hand, and said, "Thank
you for your service!" The surrounding tables got quiet as
people watched our exchange. "I would like to buy you lunch as
a way of thanking you for your service to our country." As I said
that, I put the $25 down on the table. He resisted, but I
insisted, and he smiled, and we shook hands again. I then said,
"You and your fellow soldiers are appreciated more than you
will ever know. Thank you!" and I walked away.

Again, the timing of what just happened then put me in line at
Peet's Coffee at a special time.

The young woman in front of me (who was probably about 20) was at an energy level of 5 and was spreading positivity and joy. The way she engaged the guy from the Peet's Coffee team was amazing and inspiring. She didn't just order. She didn't just say the normal "Good morning, may I have a mocha?" She poured her positivity, energy, and optimism into the barista. Here is what she said at the end of their conversation: "Thanks so much for all your help! I hope the rest of your day is amazing! You deserve it!" with a huge smile. She left the guy drastically better than she found him. I love the concept of "always leaving people better than you found them." This young lady had that nailed!

I'm normally very positive, energized, and friendly with people, but this young lady raised the bar. After I connected with the barista (I tried to match the young lady, but I may have settled for the silver medal on this one), I then saw the young lady waiting for her coffee. I decided to share my thoughts with her, but before that encounter, my negative voice tried to talk me out of it. (Are you seeing a trend?)

My negative voice started saying things like, "She is going to think you are some creepy, older, married guy," etc. But I fought off my negative voice and followed my positive voice's lead and walked right up to the young lady and said, "Excuse me. I just want to tell you that the positivity, energy, and vibe you bring to the world is inspiring. I have a young daughter, who is only four years old. But if she grows up and handles herself like you, I will be a very proud dad."

She smiled, teared up, and started to cry.

I then said, "I don't know who your parents are, but they must be remarkable!"

She then really started to cry. But they were happy tears, and she thanked me in a way that seemed so much bigger than a simple thank you. She was moved.

As we parted ways, I said, "Please tell your parents that they are remarkable and have an awesome day!" She smiled and said thank you again and walked off.

Now, the barista and the Peet's Coffee team were kind of wondering what just happened. They could tell that the discussion I just had was a positive and powerful one. I smiled as I went to grab my coffee and leave. But just as I went to step away, a guy who had just ordered came walking along. I said, "Hey! How are you?" and he said "Good! How are you?" to which I replied "Awesome!"

He smiled and kind of laughed out loud and said, "Wow! That is an amazing answer! Why are you awesome?" I then explained that I have an amazing wife, three remarkable and healthy kids, and a job I love. I have so much to be thankful for, and I'm having fun, so I'm awesome.

He then said something that surprised me. "Do you have time to sit and have coffee with me right now?"

My negative voice said, "That's strange. I should say no." But my positive voice said, "Why not?"

So, after my new friend's coffee came, we grabbed a seat. His name was Doran, and he is from Israel. He is warm, friendly, and a family man. We talked about our families, and then the discussion moved to him sharing that his mom had just passed away from cancer. I explained that I run the Boston Marathon every year to raise funds for Dana-Farber Cancer Institute, since my mom was treated there when I was a kid. I asked Doran if it would be okay to add his mom's name to the shirt I wear when I run the Boston Marathon. I always run in memory of, or in support of, hundreds of people I call "Cancer Warriors." Doran started to cry, and we shared some tears together.

The Peet's Coffee team watched as a second customer was crying after speaking with me, and I imaged them thinking, "What is this guy doing to all our customers?"

About 15 minutes into our time together, Doran asked me to explain my "Awesome!" answer at a deeper level. I explained how I had just talked about "Earning Your Awesome!" at a conference I was blessed to speak at. He then asked me to explain what I did for work besides speaking, and I told him about Breakthrough Health (the company I started in 2004) and our mission to positively impact 100 million lives by 2025.

He then said, "Have you ever thought of writing a book?"

I explained that I had published my first book in 2013, titled *The No Excuses Diet*, and that it was actually an *anti*-diet book. I also mentioned that I was working on my second book titled, *The 12 Key Habits to Thrive*.

"How did your first book do?" he asked. "Did you sell a lot of books?"

I explained how the book had ended up on the *Today Show* and hit number three on the overall Best Seller List for Amazon. Doran then gave me a huge smile and said, "Amazing!"

I shifted the conversation and asked him to tell me more about what he did for work. He had mentioned earlier in the discussion that he "had a few companies" he'd started, but he had quickly deflected the conversation back to me.

Doran said, "I will tell you more about my companies, but I want to start by explaining something interesting. One of my companies sells directly to Costco, BJ's, Target, and Walmart—including the book divisions. I know the lead book buyers at all four places, and I would like to represent your next book."

I was floored, and my jaw was on the ground. I said, "Awesome! I'm in!"

"Are you comfortable with us negotiating right now and finalizing the deal?" he asked.

I said yes, and he explained how he structured all his book partnerships with writers the same way and shared the percentages. I then replied, "That seems fair—I'm in!" and we shook hands. It was amazing!

Now I want to revisit the few things that led to this key chance encounter and meeting:

1. I had trained for my speaking event and was still at an energy level of 5 after the event.
2. I fought off my negative voice four times (to avoid the french fries, to buy the Marine lunch, to praise to the

remarkable young lady at Peet's Coffee, and to sit down for coffee with Doran).

3. I had earned my awesome so that, when Doran asked me how I was doing, I genuinely replied, "Awesome!"

4. My answer of "Awesome!" was the only reason a stranger asked to have coffee with me.

If you bought this book at Costco, BJ's, Target, or Walmart, then you can tie it back to my chance encounter with a remarkable man named Doran after earning my awesome!

Hopefully, you can now see the power of focusing on your energy. You will not only realize that you *get* to work toward your goal, but you will also feel happier and more optimistic doing so. You also never know what might happen when you listen to your positive voice and earn your awesome!

Quick Tip: Set a reminder on your phone every three hours (at 9:00 a.m., noon, 3:00 p.m., and 6:00 p.m., for example) that says, "What is your energy level?" Or possibly combine this reminder with your "Who is at the podium?" reminder. So maybe the combined reminder is "Podium/Energy?" Your negative voice may say this is nerdy, but it's highly effective.

Chapter Seven

KEY HABIT #3: CONTROL YOUR STRESS

Everyone has some amount of stress in life. The key to thriving is learning how to control stress so that it does not become overwhelming and all-consuming.

Excess stress can affect our health, our productivity, and our relationships. When we are overly stressed we have a tendency to slip back into unhealthy habits. We may overeat or drink too much. We may skip workouts or become distracted with social media when we are supposed to be working. We may become impatient with our loved ones or isolate and withdraw. With a plan in place to control stress, however, we can remain focused on our end goals and maintain our healthy habits that will allow us to thrive.

LEARN TO SAY NO

One of the best ways to decrease your stress is to start saying no to some of the pulls and requests on your time. When we say yes to too many things, we get overwhelmed, and our stress increases. There is an opportunity cost every time you say yes to a time commitment (volunteering at a school, church committee, etc.) When you overcommit, you push your own health and wellness down your priority list and hinder your ability to nail the key habits. Learning to say no (especially if you are a people pleaser) can be very challenging, but you will get more comfortable with it over time.

DIAL IN YOUR TOP 3 PRIORITIES

One way to learn to say no is to identify your top three priorities, both personally and professionally (three of each). You will then use these as your filter for deciding what you say yes or no to. If a request fits into your top three priorities, the answer is yes. If not, the answer is no. If the idea of saying no makes your skin crawl, then welcome to the "I'm Human Club." With practice though, you will get better and better at saying no.

As an example, here are my top three priorities, both personal and professional (#1 and #3 are the same for me in both categories.

MY TOP 3 PRIORITIES (PERSONALLY & PROFESSIONALLY):

1. To be the absolute best version of myself (mentally, physically, spiritually and emotionally)!
2. Personally: To support Karen, Alex, Ben and Adeline in being the absolute best versions of themselves! Professionally: To support my team in being the absolute best versions of themselves!
3. To positively impact as many people as humanly possible!

I read these three times daily to be reminded of what my priorities are.

Invest some time into identifying your top three priorities, and then use them as your filter for what you say yes or no to. You will find this challenging at first, but it will be freeing, and ultimately, will decrease your stress as you will not be over-committed.

4 KEYS TO CONQUERING STRESS

Another way to control stress is to have a simple, but impactful, process for dealing with it. That is why I came up with my 4 Keys to Conquering Stress. By using this approach, you will be able to manage stress and compartmentalize it, so it does not rob you of your happiness and health.

Here are my 4 Keys to Conquering Stress:

1. Check in about the reality of your situation. Our
    negative voices usually try to act like things are a much
    bigger deal than they probably are. This simple check-
    in enables you to get to the core of what is really going
    on. Most people eventually get to this, but only after
    wasting a lot of time.
2. Identify your actionable options. What actions are
    available for you to take to positively impact the
    situation?
3. Choose an action and take it. After you choose an
    action, don't think about it for an hour. Unless it is
    something you truly need to run by someone, or really
    feel you need additional input on, act right away. Most
    people let their negative voice talk them into holding
    off on *any* action, so they can keep stressing about it.
    Forget that! Pick an action and take it!
4. Mentally bench it. What do I mean by bench it?
    Temporarily, just for the near term, forget about it.
    You took action and, at this point, you just need to
    wait to hear back. In the meantime, clear your mind of
    thinking about it and worrying about it.

Here is how I visualize implementing the 4 Keys to Conquering
Stress: Think about a blank desk. Someone who doesn't have a
process for managing stress would have papers scattered all over
the desk. The papers represent the different things they are
stressed about.

Now compare that to someone using the 4 Keys to Conquering
Stress. Imagine they have shoe boxes lined up at the end of the

desk, and each shoe box has a label indicating various stressful situations. All the sheets for each situation are in their own box, and you just pull one box out at a time to deal with that situation. Once you have gone through the four steps, you close the box and slide it back to the end of the desk. With this approach, you have a clear desk and a clear mind.

I know this sound simple, but trust me, it works.

IT'S JUST A JOB

Many people have been fooled by their negative voice into believing their job is the most important thing in the world. Yes, we want to perform at our best and excel in our careers. We need the job to support our lives. But the irony is that, the more you make the shift toward realizing that *you* are more important, the more time you will invest in your self-care, and that, ultimately, will improve your job performance. If you do not take the time to focus on your own health and self-care, you may not be around as long as you deserve. This means you will not be able to do the work you are meant to do or to provide for any people who need you.

Please don't let your negative voice cry foul and try to fool you into thinking I'm trying to get you to quit your job. I'm not. I'm just guiding you in seeing that you can invest time each day on your self-care, to decrease stress and improve your job performance.

Make little shifts like staying hydrated, taking the stairs, parking a bit further from the door at the grocery store or office, walking in place while on the phone, doing a 15- to 30-minute daily workout, etc. These small shifts compound over time. And again, if your negative voice is trying to convince you that you can't fit this in, then please add up your TV and social media time each day, and you will probably see that you can find the 15-30 minutes.

"The graveyards of America are full of indispensable people."
— Unknown

This is a brutal quote, but it's true. When we are gone, someone else will step in. I don't point that out to demotivate you but to, hopefully, nudge you to reduce your stress when it comes to work. You deserve to be around for as long as you can. I know it can be challenging, but it is so important to find the balance between the stress of doing what we have to do to support our lives, and taking care of ourselves so that we can live a long, healthy life.

STRESS CAN LEAD TO PAYING THE ULTIMATE PRICE

In 2017, I was blessed to be a keynote speaker at a big event in California. After I finished, I was approached by a woman named Jen. She had an amazing vibe about her, and she declared that she needed, and wanted, to hire me as her Peak Performance Coach. Jen was stressed, exhausted, and wanted to drop 45 pounds. We started the next week.

Within a few years, Jen was down 38 pounds and feeling trans-formed and remarkable. She even came to one of our wellness retreats in Vermont in 2018 and then brought her husband, Pete, and her three adult sons the following summer (in 2019). After the retreat, I was given the blessing of being Pete's Peak Performance Coach, and he proceeded to drop 40 pounds over the next year.

In the spring of 2020, Jen became extremely stressed, as her industry (the mortgage industry) was going through a period of explosive growth. Throughout that spring, Jen struggled to pull back on her workload, as she juggled the impact of the pandemic and the crazy work volume.

As her coach, I tried everything possible to get her to pull back. But, as a very competitive and driven, Type A personality, nothing was working. She was then set to go on a week-long vacation with Pete and another couple they had been close friends with, and vacationing with, for 30 years.

Jen and I mapped it out that she would not work during that vacation, and I stressed the importance of her truly needing a recharge. That didn't happen.

On our first coaching call after her trip, she launched into how their friends didn't understand her and that they told her and Pete that they didn't want to vacation with them in the future. As I pressed Jen, she shared that she had worked the entire time.

By that point, I had become close friends with Jen and Pete. They were even supposed to fly out to Boston from California that prior April to stay at my house and cheer me on in the Boston Marathon (the April 2020 Boston Marathon, which ended up being postponed due to the pandemic).

After Jen admitted to me that she had worked her entire vacation, I took a risk and made the following statement to her, knowing how close she was with her late dad: "Jen, do you know how mad your dad is going to be if this stress takes you out and you walk up to him in heaven?"

She laughed it off and said she knew she needed to change. That conversation was in July of 2019.

Here is a text Jen sent me on August 9, 2019:

"So I need to fill you in.

Went to the Dr on Friday and they did an EKG. My EKG was perfect.

My blood pressure was high and has been running high around 150/97.

He wanted to put me on meds.

I said no because I know it's for the rest of my life if I do and I know it's stress and I need to get my act together.

I have taken the weekend off. Took a 4 mile walk with Pete yesterday and today. Yesterday we went to the beach and out to dinner.

Today we walked and then just relaxed, listened to music, and floated in the pool, and had 1 drink.

I just took my blood pressure. 120/81.

Time to take care of Jen and stop comparing myself to the top in the industry. Not a fair comparison until I get my team in place.

I was working, on average, 15-hour days since March with no days off and the result is great production but killing myself. 16 pounds from my low and high blood pressure.

All done with that Russian Roulette game!

Onward and upward!"

Seventeen days later, I received a call from Pete. He could barely talk, but he stated, "Jen is gone. She died of a heart attack last night. I was traveling, and she passed away at 8:30 p.m. at her desk. She worked herself to death."

Jen was only 59. She left behind her amazing husband, her three remarkable adult sons, and a world that needed her smile, her heart, and her leadership. She also left behind her future grandchildren, who deserved her.

Pete gave me permission to share Jen's story and her text, in order to, hopefully, save lives. If you have been really stressed due to your hectic job, please use Jen's story to alter your perspective. It's truly *just* a job, and your health, happiness, and life are too valuable to risk due to stress.

In closing out this chapter on controlling stress, please focus on saying no to more things and to implementing the 4 Keys to Conquering Stress. You will be pleasantly surprised how much peacefulness and joy come back into your life and how reducing your stress sets you up to thrive!

Chapter Eight

KEY HABIT #4: HAVE AN ATTITUDE OF GRATITUDE

"Happiness is letting go of what you think your life is supposed to look like and celebrating it for everything that it is." — Mandy Hale

Being grateful about everything you have is a key factor in thriving. When we are grateful, we have a better attitude and are more likely to take action on the habits that fuel good health, energy, and happiness. We are able to take more action, because being grateful puts us in a more positive state. We recognize our challenges, but we do not let them dominate our every thought. We are able to put our life in perspective, because we strive to be grateful for what we have, rather than to focus on what we do not have.

There are millions of people in this world who are suffering (they don't have housing, food, or even clean water). Don't let your negative voice tell you, "I have heard that many times before, blah, blah, blah." It's true.

Your life, and everything you have, is truly a gift, and when you view it that way, you harness emotional leverage that will be rocket fuel for taking action on the habits that lead to you achieving your goals and thriving. Plus, being grateful makes life drastically more enjoyable for you and everyone you spend time with!

> "When we change the way we look at things, the things we look at change." — Wayne Dyer

AN OLD SCHOOL WAY TO CRANK UP YOUR GRATITUDE

You heard about my mom early in the book, and she was amazing. My parents were divorced when I was only two, so my mom raised four kids on her own while working multiple jobs. We struggled financially, but the currency in our home was love, and by that measure, we were rich.

On Sundays after church, Mom would occasionally drive us into Boston (I grew up 26 miles outside of the city). Although she didn't tell us the reasoning at the time, the intention of these trips was to crank up our gratitude.

We would take her light blue 1970 Monte Carlo and drive through the projects in Boston, while Mom talked to my siblings and me about how blessed we were. She would explain how blessed we were to have a yard to play in, food in the fridge, etc. By the time we drove back into our neighborhood, our house looked like a castle, the yard was amazing, and the powdered milk and boxed mashed potatoes we had for dinner were delicious. We arrived home with attitudes of gratitude, and it changed the energy and vibe in my house.

Here is another powerful quote from my amazing mom:

> "If you have your health, someone to love, a roof over your head, and food in the fridge, then you have everything you need for an amazing life. Don't ever forget that!" — Dory Roche

USE THE PROBLEM SWAP TO CRANK UP YOUR GRATITUDE

The problem swap is an imaginary flea market, but instead of people having booths with things to sell, they have tables that have all their problems laid out. You walk into the problem swap with your problems, and you get to walk around and look at the problems other people have on their tables. If you see a set of problems someone else has, that seem better than your problems, then you can swap.

Here is the interesting thing...most people would leave again with their *own* problems. This is not to downplay your challenges. But the reality is, there are many people in this world who are dealing with truly major problems (lack of food, lack of shelter, diseases, etc.). Your negative voice can scoff at this, but it's true. Yes, we all have problems we are dealing with. Some are major and some are not. But if we compare them to the big problems others are dealing with, by using the problem swap, we will have a different perspective of the problems we have.

If you entered the problem swap, do you think you would exit with your problems? I'm guessing you would.

Being grateful is another area in which our negative or positive voice affects how we see the world. As I covered earlier in the book, our negative voices guide us to focus on what is wrong (with the world, with our jobs, with our family, with ourselves, etc.) and make us feel ungrateful. But our positive voices guide us to focus on what is right and make us feel grateful. Your decision to embrace your positive voice is going to lead to you embracing having an attitude of gratitude. That will leave you in a more positive state in which to take action on simple habits (water, sleep, nutrition, exercise, and positive content) that will fuel your pursuit of your goals and lead to thriving.

> "What you focus on expands. When you focus on the goodness in life, you create more of it." — Oprah Winfrey

USE YOUR GIFT

In the chapter on focusing on your energy, I talked about using different language to frame your attitude about any work you have to do. This ties into being grateful for what you are able to do, whatever that may be, rather than to see what you have to do as a burden.

For example, if you are currently fairly healthy, it is a gift you can be grateful for! You don't *have* to exercise; you *get* to exercise! That simple shift in mindset can be the key to reframing your daily workouts and making them more enjoyable. View what you can do as a gift!

Each year, as I run the Boston Marathon, I say to myself over and over again, "Use your gift!" I do this because the fact that I'm healthy enough to run a marathon is a blessing and a gift. I don't *have* to run the Boston Marathon each year—I *get* to.

There are many people who would give anything to be healthy enough to go for a walk or a run or to nail a workout. As you move forward, keep this in mind each day as you consider doing your workouts. You don't *have* to exercise—you *get* to! That's something to be grateful for!

In closing out this chapter on gratitude, I invite you to consider just how blessed you truly are. If we are intentional in our voice choice, and our positive voice is at the podium, then we will feel grateful about what we have and about what we can do. We will feel empowered and positive and, therefore, more prepared (and more likely) to take action on our goals. All of this is the basis of thriving.

Chapter Nine

KEY HABIT #5: UPGRADE YOUR TEAM AND EMBRACE BEING A LEADER

"The people we surround ourselves with either raise or lower our standards. They either help us to become the best version of ourselves or encourage us to become lesser versions of ourselves. We become like our friends. No man becomes great on his own. No woman becomes great on her own. The people around them help to make them great. We all need people in our lives who raise our standards, remind us of our essential purpose, and challenge us to become the best version of ourselves." — Matthew Kelly

Life is a team sport and you can't win the game playing alone! Surrounding yourself with positive, energized, and supportive people is a must and a game changer. The reason upgrading your team is a Key Habit to Thrive is because you match the healthy or unhealthy habits of your friends, and as this entire book is about, you need healthy habits to thrive.

"If you look at an individual, they are a direct reflection of the aspirations of the five people they spend the most time with."
— Tony Robbins

We think, move, talk, dream, and live like the people we hang out with.

If you hang out with negative people, with no dreams and no goals, then you will become a negative person with no dreams and no goals. But, fortunately, the opposite is also true. If you hang out with positive and energized people, with big dreams and huge goals, you will become a positive and energized person with big dreams and huge goals.

The following quote is another way to look at this—we want to be the man or women in the arena, not the one in the stands watching:

"It's not the critic who counts; not the man who points out how the strong man stumbles, or where the doer of deeds could have done them better. The credit belongs to the man who is actually in the arena, whose face is marred by dust and sweat and blood; who strives valiantly; who errs, who comes short again and again, because there is no effort without error and shortcoming; but who does actually strive to do the deeds; who knows great enthusiasms, the great devotions; who spends himself in a worthy cause; who at the best knows in the end the triumph of high achievement, and who at the worst, if he fails, at least fails while daring greatly, so that his place shall never be with those cold and timid souls who neither know victory nor defeat." — Theodore Roosevelt

MINIMIZE YOUR EXPOSURE TO NEGATIVE PEOPLE AND SURROUND YOURSELF WITH POSITIVE PEOPLE

Most likely, you are surrounded by a variety of people. As you work toward thriving, it is important to start to notice the kind of people you are spending time with. Are you surrounded by more negative people or positive people?

Negative people drain the energy out of us. They talk about how tough everything is, how unhappy they are, and how difficult life is—and most of the time, they drag us down with them. We all have bad days, but you need to be careful about spending too much time with negative people who take you in the wrong direction. I'm very guarded about letting people drag me down, and you should be as well.

As you start to take on new, healthy habits you may feel that some people in your world are trying to drag you in the wrong direction. This isn't because they don't care about you; it's because your healthy choices can make them feel uncomfortable. As spectators, the fact that they are not achieving their potential becomes painfully evident as they watch your rocket leave the pad. When people see others thriving (especially successfully losing weight), they start asking themselves tough questions like "How come I'm not doing that?" This leads to feelings of insecurity and generates negative comments.

It's critical that you communicate to your friends, family, and coworkers how important your new, healthy habits are to you. Have a few simple conversations about how you need your support network to stay positive and to encourage you. You will protect your progress by being vocal about your needs.

Sometimes, the people in our lives will try to discourage us from making healthy changes, setting big goals, and trying to thrive. If we listen to the family members, friends, neighbors, and coworkers who doubt us, then we will never accomplish anything! When you talk about walking your first 5K, losing 40 pounds, or going for that big job promotion, people sometimes get uncomfortable and react by trying to talk you out of chasing down your goals. As I mentioned earlier, many times these people are dealing with their own insecurities, and their comments are not truly about you. It is important to stay true to your plan and your goals, despite any feedback you get from others.

If I had listened to the doubters when I weighed 224 pounds and was wearing size 38 pants, and decided not to run my first Boston Marathon back in 1995, I would not be who I am or where I am today. No matter what anyone around you thinks or says, you can accomplish anything you set your mind to. You just need to take it one step at a time, stay consistent with your plan, and keep it fun.

This same advice applies to situations with family members and close friends. Getting together with family or friends during the holidays or other events is usually fun. But when your mom, aunt, sister, or friend starts making negative comments about the weight you have lost, it can turn a fun time into an uncomfortable one very quickly. The best advice I can give you is to kill them with kindness, with replies like, "I'm actually doing this the healthy way, by exercising and eating right. And the great thing is, I'm having fun, and I feel amazing."

If killing them with kindness doesn't work, you may have to resort to a firmer response, such as, "If you don't have anything nice to say about my weight loss, then please don't comment on it." You've worked too hard and come too far to let anyone rain on your parade. Again, you need to stay true and committed to your plan.

Positive people, on the other hand, focus on and talk about what is right (in the world, with their families, with their jobs and with themselves), what they are reading and learning, and fun opportunities for growth. They compliment you on your hard work and encourage you to stick to your plan. They ask you questions about your journey and share your excitement in what you have accomplished.

You usually leave conversations with positive people feeling better than when you started. In fact, every interaction we have with people involves an energy exchange.

Let's look at an example. On a scale of zero to five, where five is extremely positive and zero is extremely negative, if you and I get together when you are a five and I am a one, then, by the end of our talk, we are both threes. You lifted me up, and I dragged you down. This is why surrounding ourselves with positive people is important. You are working on strengthening your own positive voice, and you are trying to focus on your energy as you work toward thriving. You need people to meet you where you are and to help raise you up, not to bring you down.

IS IT TIME FOR A FRIENDS UPGRADE?

Unfortunately, sometimes you are going to need to make the tough decision about friends who only drag you down, behave negatively, and don't embrace the new you. This is tough, but it's sometimes best to move on. I'm not telling you to forget those friends entirely, but I am asking you to be guarded about allowing people to stop you from becoming who you deserve to be.

I want to illustrate this key concept with a story:

In the late '90s, after I had lost 40 pounds and had run a few Boston Marathons, my "friends" would continually harass me about being "Mr. Fitness" or "Mr. Energy." They meant well, but after trying to deflect their comments, and, eventually, even having the tough "if you're not going to say anything positive, don't say anything at all" conversations, they kept at it.

We had all rented a house on Nantucket for a week, and the first night my friends partied, got drunk, and, as usual, were self-destructive. In the morning, I got up early and went for a ten-mile run along on the water. I felt amazing, and I was on fire when I got back to the house. My "friends" were all hungover, and they literally could not let it go that "Mr. Fitness" had run ten miles while they were all sleeping.

This went on all day and night. That night I hit my breaking point. I left the bar early, went home, and went to bed. The next morning, I got up, packed my bags, told my soon-to-be-former "friends" that I'd had enough, and I was leaving. I got a cab, hopped on a ferry, and on day three of our week-long (and expensive) vacation, I was out of there.

That decision proved to be one of the best decisions of my life, because, over the next one to three years, I went through a significant friend upgrade, from people who put me down to people who encouraged and supported me. Not surprisingly, my own life (both personally and professionally) soared!

I now have very high standards when it comes to my friends and associations. I had friends in the past who were negative, and I set them free. Why? Because I want to be around positive people, who are fired up to learn, grow, serve others, and make a positive impact on the world.

Here is another important thing to consider: As you raise your standards on the type of people you want to be friends with and associate with, you show the people in your life (especially your kids, if you have them) how to take that action. Through showing them the positive impact it has on your life, you set the example for them to evaluate their relationships as well.

HOW TO EVALUATE YOUR RELATIONSHIPS

As you begin to evaluate your relationships with the people in your life, here is one key question to help guide you: Does the person get as excited, or more excited, than you when you share a crazy goal or win with them? If so, that is a great sign. If not, you may want to consider moving on. You deserve to have energized, positive, growth-minded, and happy friends and associations!

One of the quickest ways to meet and develop friendships and associations with these types of people is to get your energy level up to a 5 (or at least a 4) and keep it there. Why is that important? Because most people bond with other people at the same energy level. Groups of 4s or 5s are not interested in hanging out with 1s or 2s, because they drag us down.

Don't let your negative voice cry foul on this—it's the truth. If you want to upgrade your friends and associations, upgrade your energy to a 4 or 5. The 4s and 5s are Doers (versus Talkers), and they are inspiring and fun to be around.

HAVING TROUBLE FINDING YOUR TEAM? START ONE!

If you are having trouble finding a group of positive friends or associations, it is never too late to start one!

Mary is one of my Peak Performance Coaching clients, and she is in the UK. About six months after the beginning of the 2020 "health situation" (this is the term I use instead of the coronavirus), we were talking through the importance of surrounding ourselves with positive people. She was having a difficult time finding a group, given all of the social restrictions. I suggested to her that she start a virtual book group and use Zoom, with the intention of changing to an in-person group after the health situation ended. She invited eight people, seven accepted, and they have been meeting monthly and having a blast. It has been, and continues to be, amazing for Mary and her friends to connect with positive, energized, and like-minded people.

I have also been fortunate enough to create a group of my own. Even though I have been part of a dynamic group of world-class business leaders and CEOs since 2013, I wanted to find an additional group of leaders, who were fully committed to being World-Class Guides. To me, a World-Class Guide is someone who has scaled the Peak Performance Ladder to live and be at a World-Class level, and is now focused on helping others move up the ladder in their personal and professional lives. In essence, it is someone who is thriving and is committed to helping others thrive. You can learn about the Peak Performance Ladder and being a World-Class Guide by going to www.12KeyHabits.com/PeakLadder. After searching and having trouble finding that type of team of people, I decide to start it myself.

In September 2021, I hosted a group of world-class people at my special place in Vermont for the 1st Annual Positive Impact Summit! The goal of the Positive Impact Summit is for the participants to share ideas, strategies, and tools that enable us to positively impact and serve more people and accelerate our positive impact.

I identified ten attributes for the people I invited to my 1st Annual Positive Impact Summit:

1. Positive
2. Energetic (energy level of 5)
3. Grateful
4. Healthy (at goal weight or dropping 1–2 pounds per week)
5. Growth-oriented (a student of personal and

professional development—reading books, watching videos, etc.)

6. Service-oriented (constantly trying to serve and improve others)
7. World-Class (World-Class Level or higher on the Peak Performance Ladder, or on track to be there within one year)
8. Humble
9. A track record of excellence, service and impact
10. Impeccable character

At the Positive Impact Summit, each attendee presents for 30–60 minutes and covers three key questions:

1. What is the most important lesson you have ever learned, and who taught it to you?
2. What is the most important book you have ever read, and what did it teach you?
3. What is the most important habit you have implemented in your life, and how has it impacted you?

The intention was that the three-day event would be one of the most fun and impactful experiences of our lives, and it was. In fact, 13 of the 16 participants are hosting their own Positive Impact Summits in 2022. Plus, all 16 are coming back in 2022, in addition to 24 new invitees for this year's event.

I have a suggestion that may sound "too big" for your negative voice. Why don't you start your own Positive Impact Summit (either in person or on Zoom)? Maybe it isn't three days long—maybe it is one day, or even three hours. The duration is not important. All that matters is that you get positive and like-minded people together to share, bond, grow, and serve at a greater level.

Maybe you don't end up launching a book group like Mary or a Positive Impact Summit like I did. All that matters is that you find friends and associations who lift you up, inspire you to grow personally and professionally, and lead to you being a better version of yourself.

EMBRACE BEING A LEADER

Viewing yourself as a leader is a key move to thrive in your life! This is because you will want to put in more effort to stay positive, be healthy, and lead by example, so that others (especially family members) can use you as a role model for what is possible.

My definition of a leader is anyone who is in a position to be watched and followed by others. That means that you are already a leader. You have the potential of being watched and followed during any interaction you have with others. Don't let your negative voice paint this as a bad thing or something to stress about. I'm simply guiding you on adding more motivation to take action on the healthy habits (water, sleep, nutrition, exercise, and positive content) that fuel you being the best leader possible. You have been a leader for decades, and it's time to embrace that role and thrive!

LEADERSHIP IS NEEDED NOW MORE THAN EVER

During calm waters, leaders are watched by others. But during stormy waters (like in the middle of a pandemic), people *study* leaders.

Here is an example: If you are flying on a plane and you run into serious turbulence, you do two things. You check your seatbelt and then you look for a flight attendant. You look for him or her to get reassurance of just how bad the turbulence is. If she is still talking about her grandchildren with the people two rows up, that is reassuring. But if she is speed walking up the aisle, it makes you nervous that this is serious turbulence.

The same thing happens during other challenging times. You are being studied, and it's time to embrace that opportunity to lead, serve and thrive.

Your negative voice may be trying to complain and say, "What does leadership have to do with thriving?" As I explained above, you are a leader, and embracing that role will lead to you paying more attention to the health habits (water, sleep, nutrition, exercise, and positive content) that fuel energy, positivity, health, and, ultimately, thriving. That will then inspire others (family, friends, coworkers, etc.) to elevate themselves and follow your lead.

By the way, one of the most important reasons to crank your energy level up to 5 each day is so that you have additional capacity to lead and serve. As I mentioned earlier in the book, you can't give away what you don't have. Prior to the health situation, I had been telling people for years to train for life's big moments in advance. I would talk about how you can't build a sword and armor in the middle of a battle. When the health situation hit, most people didn't have the energy and health reserves built up and were not ready to lead and serve. That has led to a lot of people not having the mental, physical, spiritual, and emotional endurance to get through these trying times.

Embrace being a leader so that you can guide your family, friends, coworkers, and even strangers, through calm and stormy waters. By upgrading your team and embracing your leadership, you will make huge progress as you work toward your goals and start to thrive!

Chapter Ten

KEY HABIT #6: EMBRACE BEING YOUR OWN EFFORT-BASED HEAD COACH

In February of 2014, I was blessed to attend a conference, and one of the keynote speakers was the thought leader in the Science of Behavioral Change, Dr. James Prochaska. The Science of Behavioral Change is just a fancy way of explaining how to establish good habits or beat bad habits.

Dr. Prochaska is the creator of the 6 Stages of Behavioral Change that have been used for many decades by AA, the American Cancer Society, and by the National Institute of Health for many of their change-modification programs.

When it comes to trying to beat a disempowering habit (like eating too many desserts, overeating in general, drugs, alcohol, etc.) or establishing an empowering habit (like daily workouts, skipping desserts, getting seven hours of sleep, etc.), Dr. Prochaska is the guy! So, when I received an email a few months prior to the conference, asking if I wanted to attend a day early and spend the day with Dr. Prochaska and a small group, I was all in.

That day with Dr. Prochaska turned into one of the most valuable and impactful days of my professional life. It ended up being just Dr. Prochaska, his wife, Janice (who is also a behavioral scientist), me, and eleven health insurance executives. It was just the fourteen of us, for about six hours, and it was powerful.

At one point, Dr. Prochaska asked us what we thought the number one factor is for an individual to beat a disempowering habit or establish an empowering habit. We gave him every answer imaginable, and he would say the same thing each time: "That is a great guess, but that is not it!"

He then made the following statement: After over 40 years of studying people and their efforts to change, the number one factor that will determine their success is belief from their coach!

Wow! That was shocking and exciting. At the next break, I rushed up to Dr. Prochaska and said, "Dr. Prochaska, that was amazing! Would you please tell me if the following is accurate? My company provides live-streamed and recorded workout videos, plus we offer 1-on-1 coaching and group coaching. Is it accurate for us to assume the head coaching role for our clients, as we empower them, but, ultimately, for them to take over as their *own* health coach, with us becoming, really, like their assistant coaches?"

Dr. Prochaska smiled and nodded. "That is correct!"

So, what does that mean? It means that you are your own head coach. If you feel like you are not where you want to be in life, it is probably because your coach has been your negative voice. She or he talks down to you, treats you as if you are not enough, and is generally disempowering. No wonder you have not been able to thrive! You have been set up to fail by not having a coach who believes in you and that coach is your own negative voice!

That is the bad news. Are you ready for the good news? I'm already guiding you in this book toward elevating your positive voice to be your head coach. Your positive voice believes in you, knows you are already world-class, and is 100% confident that you can and will achieve your goals. How fun is that to think about?

You now know exactly why you have struggled with meeting goals, whether that be weight loss or career- or relationship-based goals, and you now know how to fix it for good.

Here is something important to keep in mind as you embrace being your own head coach: You lose the built-in excuse for why it didn't work. Many people will play the blame game when they don't drop the weight, get the promotion, or thrive. They blame their coach or the program. But the reality is, they are their own head coach, and with that ownership comes responsibility. Is this scary? Yes. But when was the last time you did something great in your life without being scared? The answer is probably never.

Ditch your negative voice's guidance on playing the blame game. Instead, embrace being your own head coach, and then guide yourself (through controlling the podium of your mind and through the other 11 Key Habits found in this book) to thrive.

One additional point: If you don't currently believe in yourself, then I suggest borrowing belief from one of your biggest fans. The people who love us are our biggest fans. They get as excited, or even more excited, than we do when something amazing happens, and they have our backs when things go wrong. They also believe in us, and you can feel it when you are with them. These fans may be your spouse, best friend, coach, or sister.

If you currently don't have a biggest fan to borrow self-belief from, then I suggest you look back to a time in your life when you had a coach, boss, coworker, or friend who *did* believe in you. Harness the power of those positive memories and that belief and use it now to take action on your self-care.

My mom was my biggest fan, and I used her belief in me (and her continual reminders to believe in myself) to push forward (both for the 12 years I had her and ever since).

Here is a powerful quote from my mom:

> "You can be anything you want to be if you believe in yourself, treat people right, work really hard, and always do the right thing." — Dory Roche

It's time for you to embrace being your own head coach and to believe in yourself! And for your positive voice to be that coach! Once you accept and embrace this and act upon it (along with the other 11 Key Habits to Thrive), your rocket will leave the pad.

EMBRACE BEING AN EFFORT-BASED COACH

Now that you are taking over as your own head coach and inviting your positive voice to guide you, it's time to make a second important and impactful decision. It's time to shift from being a results-based coach to an effort-based coach!

Most people are results-based coaches. Often, especially with weight loss, it is all about results! If you don't drop weight, then you are not successful. It doesn't matter if your energy is up, or your vibe is improving, or you have stopped yelling at your kids. If the scale shows a number that is the same as last week—or a *higher* number—then you failed. This thinking and this approach is due to your now-former head coach—your negative voice.

A key part of your life-altering transition from your negative voice being your coach to your positive voice being your coach is embracing being an effort-based coach. An effort-based coach is focused only on effort and doesn't judge or worry about the results. By putting 100% of your focus into your effort, you harness all your energy into action and drastically improve your results. Plus, being an effort-based coach is about 100 times more fun than being a results-based coach.

I love the following quote from one of the top American runners in history, Steve Prefontaine:

"To give anything less than your best is to sacrifice the gift."

Our best looks different on any given day, so don't let your negative voice interpret this quote as you needing to be perfect. Perfectionism imprisons many people, as it's unrealistic and only leads to a feeling of being less than. The goal is to simply do the best you can each day. Some days you are on fire and nailing your habits. Other days you are off (maybe you didn't sleep well), and your best may be nailing your hydration and fueling your body properly. The key is to be kind to yourself— you wouldn't expect perfection from anyone else, so why would you allow your negative voice to convince you that perfectionism is the goal? Let's end that as of now!

While we are ditching perfectionism, let's also ditch all-or-nothing thinking. We are all human, and we make mistakes and get off course. The best thing to do in that situation is to simply jump back in and take action on your healthy habits (water, sleep, nutrition, exercise, and positive content).

Two of the greatest coaches in the history of sports are John Wooden and Nick Saban, who are both effort-based coaches. Coach Wooden won ten national championships while coaching the UCLA men's basketball team, and Nick Saban has won seven national championships as the coach of Alabama's football team. They lead and focus their teams on their effort and on taking consistent action on the key habits that lead to success. When Coach Wooden coached, and while Coach Saban coaches, their athletes aren't worried about being chewed out about losing a game. All that matters is effort. The following quotes are some of my favorite and are at the heart of being your own effort-based head coach.

"The goal in life is the same as in basketball: make the effort to do the best you are capable of doing—in marriage, at your job, in the community, for your country. Make the effort to contribute in whatever way you can. You may do it materially or with time, ideas, or work." — John Wooden

"Success comes from knowing that you did your best to become the best that you are capable of becoming." — John Wooden

"Focus on the progress, not the results." — Nick Saban

"Live by the creed that a strong work ethic, playing by the rules, and doing things the right way will bring about opportunities for success and, ultimately, happiness." — Nick Saban

"Becoming a champion is not an easy process... It is done by focusing on what it takes to get there and not on getting there." — Nick Saban.

From today onward, embrace being your own effort-based head coach. Believe in yourself. Hold yourself accountable through making a plan and working on these 12 Habits to Thrive. Focus on your effort, not just results. Celebrate progress toward your goals, but also be forgiving of yourself for any missteps. Keep doing your best to win at your game. These moves alone have the potential to be life-altering, so go for it!

Chapter Eleven

KEY HABIT #7: EXERCISE AND BE A RANDOM ACTS OF FITNESS MACHINE

A key theme of this book is that health is a foundational component of being able to thrive. It is only through actively working on your health that you will be able to have the positive energy, mood, and stamina it takes to thrive.

Exercise plays a huge role in maintaining a healthy lifestyle. While this can seem daunting to some, especially those who have struggled to make health and fitness a major part of their lives, it will be reassuring to know that exercise does not have to take up large chunks of your time. When you understand the overall benefits of exercise and then pair that with the knowledge that there are many ways to define a workout, you will realize that you can nail this key habit!

In this chapter I will explain why exercise is important, discuss the importance of sweating (working hard!), discuss the best way to exercise to get the most out of your time, and then end with a way to fit exercise into your life that will make it easier to get in all the movement you need.

ENERGY UP, MOOD UP

One of the greatest benefits of exercise is that you can significantly increase your energy and elevate your mood. In fact, I think the best reward for staying consistent with your workouts is the earned increase in energy level. Yes, fitting into smaller jeans, or losing weight, is nice. But feeling like you have enough energy to jump through the roof is the real reward.

I do have one caveat: when you start an exercise program, you might have *less* energy than usual. This is simply because your body needs to adapt to having to work harder than it is used to. But don't let the one to two weeks of decreased energy force you to associate exercise with *robbing* yourself of energy. Look at it like taking two steps back to eventually take ten steps forward.

If you don't start feeling like you have more energy from your new habit of consistent exercise after about two weeks, then please consider the following:

1. Are you doing too much (too many workouts and/or exercising too hard or long)?
2. Are you sleeping enough?
3. Are you eating enough calories and staying hydrated throughout the day?

Another benefit of exercise is that it can elevate your mood and make you feel good. Instead of looking at exercise as something you have to do to lose weight, look at it as your "attitude adjuster" and the number one way to feel better!

I saw my friend, Jim (who is 77 years young), at the fitness club after one of his daily swims. He was glowing, and was in his usual positive spirits. When I asked him how his swim was, he said, "I feel 77 years old when I start and 30 when I finish!" Then he added, "There's no medication on this planet that can give me what I get out of my exercise."

Think about this for a minute. There is no better way to beat the aging process and no better way to lift your spirits, energy, and mood than with exercise.

Like everyone, I have times when I feel overwhelmed, irritable, and don't feel like working out. Sometimes it seems easier to skip exercise so that I can get more work done. I know, however, that I always feel ten times better after a workout. I know it is worth the time it takes to get in movement.

As I have said, the person who finishes a workout is always a much more energetic, positive, and happy person than the one who started it. Instead of looking at your workouts as burdens to check off your to-do list look at them as energy and mood boosters!

A third benefit of exercise is that it is the quickest, cheapest, and simplest way to reduce stress. In fact, the more stressed you are, the more you should focus on nailing your workouts. Even though you may not feel up to a workout, think of it as an investment in your health.

Physical activity can help to take your mind off of your stressors. When you can focus on moving your body, it takes the focus off of your mind. Even a 5-minute walk can clear your head and make you feel better.

So make exercise your number one tool to raise your energy, improve your mood, and fight stress. You and your health are worth it!

Is your negative voice trying to talk you out of the exercise habit before you even start? If so, I want to point out something important. Even 10-minute workouts are fantastic and will alter your energy and vibe. You can increase that to 15 or 20 minutes, and then eventually 30 minutes, per day. But give yourself the freedom of starting slow so that you get hooked on feeling better and so that your workouts don't feel like a part-time job.

SWEATING TO FEEL GREAT

There's something powerful and empowering about sweating. It tells you that you're working hard enough and lets you know you're getting the most out of your workout. I see a lot of people at gyms doing cardio, and yet they're either not sweating or are barely sweating at all. That's a missed opportunity. The unfortunate thing is, many of them will eventually quit on themselves and their workouts because they are "not getting results," even though they're putting in the time.

Solution: Learn to love sweat! It can actually feel good. Sweat is your reward for working hard. It shows that you're working at a moderate-to-high intensity and, therefore, maximizing your fitness and weight-loss results. Although any movement (whether you're sweating or not) is great for your health, you might as well maximize your results while working out. So sweating is the way to go!

One important thing to note, that common saying in fitness, "no pain, no gain"...it isn't true! You should never be in pain during or after working out. Yes, you should sweat and test yourself, and you should be aware, later in the day and the next day, that you exercised. It's okay to feel some soreness, but you shouldn't have pain. Working out to a level where you're in pain increases your risk of injury and burnout and will most likely leave you feeling demoralized.

Instead of saying "no pain, no gain," try this affirmation to encourage yourself along the way: "No sweat, I am not there yet!"

Unless you're within two weeks of starting to exercise, or your doctor has instructed you to take it easy, then you should be sweating during your workouts in order to maximize your results. As I said above, sweating is the sign that you're working hard (not to a level of pain, but making a solid effort) and helps you maximize your calorie burning and overall results. So, when you're doing your workouts, push yourself until you sweat, and be proud!

QUALITY OVER QUANTITY IN EXERCISE

Are you doing *quality* workouts, or are you just going through the motions and "putting in your time?" Spending big chunks of time exercising is zero fun and robs you of time you could spend playing with your family, reading a book, relaxing, or doing something else you love. When the quality of your workouts is high, and you're maximizing your results, you don't have to exercise for more than 30 minutes per day. Doing quality workouts enables you to avoid feeling like exercising is a part-time job and keeps it fun. You maximize your results in quick windows of time and know that every minute invested is a step in the right direction, allowing you to crank up your energy and improve your health.

The best way to get in a quality workout is to do interval training.

INTERVAL TRAINING/WORKOUTS

During an interval workout, you will increase and decrease your exertion levels several times during your routine. You will strive for progressively higher levels of perceived exertion or heart rate for several minutes at a time. In between these "push periods," you will have 1- or 2-minute periods of recovery.

Pushing your effort level up and down taxes your body and causes it to work harder and burn more calories than exercising at one set level. Also, by adding the rest periods in between, you're able to exercise at a higher level during the push intervals and, therefore, burn more calories than you would by staying at one set pace for an extended period of time. In fact, interval workouts not only help you burn 30% more calories per workout (versus exercising at a set pace), but they also leave your metabolism elevated for up to 12 hours after each workout!

Intervals also strengthen your heart and lungs and improve your recovery rates (how quickly your heart rate drops after exertion). So, even if you are not trying to lose weight, intervals are a great way to improve your heart health and increase your overall fitness.

The great thing about interval workouts is that you can do them anywhere (in your living room, outside, or at a gym), and when doing any activity you want—all that matters is that you hit the target levels. You can do intervals by running, biking, swimming, using cardio equipment in a gym, or walking outside. You can walk up and down the stairs in your home, jump rope with your kids, have a dance party in your living room, or do an arms-only boxing workout while sitting in a chair.

You should choose activities or movement that you like to do. You will remain committed longer if you enjoy what you are doing. It is also okay to vary the types of exercise that you do too. You may go for a walk one day, dance the next day, and ride a stationary bike another day.

The key is to increase your heart rate and then let it recover (decrease). Repeat this several times over 30 minutes, and you will have completed a quality interval workout!

Some examples of what you could do for an interval workout are:

- Walk at a quick pace for three minutes, walk at a slower pace for one minute, walk at a quick pace for three minutes, walk at a slower pace for one minute. Try to increase your pace a little during each push period.
- Dance in your living room, getting your heart rate up for three minutes. Then march slowly in place for one minute to recover. Repeat this pattern.
- While sitting in a chair, move your arms in a punching movement for two minutes. Then slowly move your arms in circles for one minute to recover. Repeat."

Most people do "steady-state" exercise. Steady-state exercise is working up to a certain level of exertion and then staying there for an extended period of time. For example, someone who gets on a treadmill and walks at a pace of 3.5 mph for an hour, or someone who gets on a bike and rides at the same pace for 30 minutes, is doing steady-state training. Of course, this is better than not working out at all, but it isn't the most effective way to maximize your results.

I lost 40 pounds 26 years ago and have kept it off doing intervals. Plus, intervals are at the core of why I've been able to start and finish 12 Ironman triathlons and 27 straight Boston Marathons without hammering my body or training obsessively.

INTERVAL WORKOUTS IN THE PRESS

The power of interval training has received a lot of positive press. Here are some excerpts from three articles on the topic:

ARTICLE #1: MAYO CLINIC: "REV UP YOUR WORKOUT WITH INTERVAL TRAINING"

"Once the domain of elite athletes, interval training has become a powerful tool for the average exerciser, too."

"It's not as complicated as you might think. Interval training is simply alternating bursts of intense activity with intervals of lighter activity."

"You'll burn more calories. The more vigorously you exercise, the more calories you'll burn—even if you increase intensity for just a few minutes at a time."

To read the full article go to www.12KeyHabits.com/Intervals.

ARTICLE #2: CONSUMER REPORTS: "INTERVAL TRAINING: MORE BENEFIT, LESS FATIGUE"

"The interval method—applicable to virtually any aerobic activity and an option on most exercise machines—avoids long periods of strenuous exercise."

"That 30 percent increase in calories burned using the interval method is roughly the equivalent of exercising 30 percent longer at the original pace."

To read the full article go to www.12KeyHabits.com/Intervals.

ARTICLE #3: ASSOCIATED PRESS: "INTERVAL TRAINING CAN CUT EXERCISE HOURS SHARPLY"

"People who complain they have no time to exercise may soon need another excuse."

"High-intensity interval training is twice as effective as normal exercise," said Jan Helgerud, an exercise expert at the Norwegian University of Science and Technology. "This is like finding a new pill that works twice as well...We should immediately throw out the old way of exercising."

To read the full article go to www.12KeyHabits.com/Intervals.

30 MINUTES, 3 DAYS PER WEEK

You should do three 30-minute interval workouts each week on non-consecutive days. The reason you should only be doing three intervals per week is because your heart is a muscle, and it needs recovery time to get stronger.

Let me explain with an example: When you work a muscle, you aren't getting any stronger *during* the exercise. The muscle fibers are torn during the exercise, and then they rebuild and get stronger over the 24 to 48 hours *after* the workout. This is when the strength of the muscle increases. If you did bicep curls every day, all you would do is perpetually exhaust your bicep muscles. The same principle applies to your heart muscle. You need to give it rest every other day.

We often think that, if a little bit of something is helpful, more must be better. But, in this case, it isn't true. It may also be a new idea for some of you that you "only" need to exercise for 30 minutes each time. Some people are used to having to spend an hour or more at the gym to feel like they had a good workout. Having to commit to this length of time daily is not sustainable for most people. Thirty minutes can seem much more manageable, and it can pack in the same benefits as a longer workout.

In fact, in a study of 416,000 people over a 13-year period, researchers found that doing just *15 minutes* of moderate exercise a day is beneficial. It may add three years to your life! There is now solid research to support the notion that every step counts, and doing even 15 minutes of exercise daily is beneficial from a health standpoint. (To read the full article about this amazing research, go to www.12KeyHabits.com/15Minutes.)

Here's something amazing to consider: If exercising for 15 minutes per day can add three years to your life, what can 30 minutes per day do?

THE POWER OF USING A HEART RATE MONITOR

A heart rate monitor is a device that you wear that measures your heart rate. It is almost like having a "coach on your wrist."

A heart rate monitor gives you real-time information about how hard you are working. It allows you to be more intentional with your interval workouts, since you can use exact numbers for increasing your heart rate during pushes and letting it drop during recovery times.

Using a heart rate monitor replaces guesses about your effort level with facts. It guides you in making sure you're working out hard enough and guards you from pushing yourself too hard, risking injury and burnout in the process.

If you do not have a heart rate monitor, you can still do interval workouts using "perceived exertion." Perceived exertion uses a scale to rate your effort and your recovery. For example, on a scale of 1-10, 1 is that you are sitting on the couch and 10 is that you passed out from working too hard. Don't ever get to a 10!

An example of a 30-minute interval workout would be:

- 5 min warm-up – reach a perceived exertion of 3
- 3 min – push to perceived exertion 5
- 2 min – recover to a perceived exertion 3
- 3 min – push to perceived exertion 6
- 2 min – recover to perceived exertion 3
- 3 min – push to perceived exertion 7
- 2 min – recover to perceived exertion 3
- 3 min – push to perceived exertion 8
- 2 min – recover to perceived exertion 3
- 5 min cool-down – perceived exertion 3

If you had a heart rate monitor, you would be able to go through the same workout, but you could use your real heart rate numbers. A heart rate monitor will multiply the effectiveness of your routine since it gives you more accurate information.

Here is the order of least to most effective ways to maximize your fitness and weight-loss results:

1. Do any movement.
2. Do intervals using perceived exertion.
3. Do intervals using a heart rate monitor.
4. Do personalized intervals (based on your personal health and fitness level) using a heart rate monitor.

I want you to win by maximizing every minute of every workout you do! Take it from me, using a heart rate monitor is the way to go.

For more guidance on how to do interval workouts, please join me and 14 other world-class coaches as we lead a variety of 20-30 minute workouts that you can do at home. As of early 2022, there are 30 workouts that are streamed live each week in addition to 11,000 recorded workouts. Most of these workouts require no equipment and are for all exercise levels. We also offer workouts for indoor cycling, free weights, yoga, etc. All of these workouts will guide your effort level using perceived exertion and heart rate. If you decide to invest in a heart rate monitor, the software will help to personalize your interval workouts based on your own heart rate. Please visit EnergyUP.co to join for free!

WHY STRENGTH TRAINING IS SO IMPORTANT

In addition to workouts that get your heart rate up, workouts that focus on building strength are a big part of a healthy workout plan. You should incorporate three strength-training workouts each week, on the days that you are not doing an interval workout.

Some benefits you can expect from a strength-training program are the ability to:

- Fight off osteoporosis
- Avoid injuries (especially back injuries)
- Improve your posture
- Burn more calories at rest
- Tone your body

I developed what I call the "No Excuses Workout" to incorporate into any healthy lifestyle. This workout involves strength training using only your body weight. You do not need to go to a gym, and you do not need any equipment. This is why it is called "No Excuses" — because there are none!

The No Excuses Workout is made up of a series of squats, lunges, push-ups, sit-ups, and other strength-training movements that use only your body weight. You can find videos of these workouts (for free) by joining www.EnergyUP.co.

Another really important component of a healthy body is a healthy core. Core strengthening exercises can be done in between your interval training days as part of No Excuses Workouts (strength training).

Having a strong core is important for many reasons beyond looking good. It helps you:

- Avoid injury
- Protect your back
- Maintain good posture
- Perform better in everyday activities and sports

By consistently doing the No Excuses Workout, you'll build a strong core that will help you be safer and remain pain-free, while making you proud of your toned midsection.

BE A RANDOM ACTS OF FITNESS MACHINE

A common attribute of consistently healthy people is that they add a lot of random movement into their day. They use what I call "random acts of fitness." They sneak fitness into their lives by doing things that are not normally considered workouts. They park farther away from the store in order to get in more steps. They take the stairs instead of the elevator. They march in place while brushing their teeth. They walk around their home or office while on the phone. They have random dance parties in their kitchen while waiting for dinner to cook.

There are lots of small ways to sneak movement into your daily life. Some of it can be really fun! Remember, every step counts, and all movement increases our energy and mood, it all adds up.

WHAT IS A WORKOUT?

A lot of people think they've only done a workout if they've done at least 30 minutes of difficult exercise. That's not true! Part of the reason I've been able to keep 40 pounds off for 26 years is because I have redefined the term workout.

I consider a workout to be anything that gets your heart rate up or works your muscles more than sitting in a chair.

Here are a few examples:

1. March in place while brushing your teeth in the morning and evening. Twice a day for two to three minutes equals four to six minutes of exercise.
2. Take an extra trip to the mailbox and back when you grab your mail. You may look strange to your neighbors, but who cares, if it helps you feel amazing and thrive?
3. Take the stairs at work, the mall, or whenever you normally would take an elevator.
4. Park in the farthest spot from the door in the lot at your office, grocery store, or mall.
5. Walk up and down your stairs (or march in place) during the commercials while watching TV. The average one-hour show has 17 minutes of commercials, so moving during commercials is a great way to improve your health and stay active.

I often do a 4-minute workout in my kitchen at night by marching in place while filling up my water bottles and making my lunch for the next day. Strange? Yes. But also effective! All you need to do is be creative about what things you can do to get your heart rate up and work your muscles.

As you can see from my examples above, you can turn some of your house projects and routines into workouts and create a true win-win scenario. So be creative, and you'll be pleasantly surprised how active you are and how consistent you are with your workouts.

As you now know, you don't have to go to a gym to fit in extra workouts during the day. All you need to do is either get your heart rate up or work your muscles a little more than usual, and you're definitely doing a workout. Add random acts of fitness into this equation and you will greatly increase your health benefits.

To help you get going, I want you to make your own list of at least five ways you can add random acts of fitness to your life. Once you start adding these into your routine, they'll become habit, and you'll be amazed by the effect they can have. This extra daily movement is not only good for you, but also sends a positive signal to your brain that your health is important and is a top priority.

The base plan to thrive and meet your health goals, including reaching your goal weight, is to complete three 30-minute interval workouts and three 30-minute No Excuses Workouts (strength training) each week. Random acts of fitness are the bonus with huge payoffs! If you combine this habit with the mental habits discussed in this book, you will be well on your way to thrive.

Chapter Twelve

KEY HABIT #8: FORM YOUR LIFESTYLE/CAREER AROUND YOUR WELLNESS

Health and wellness are the basis for thriving, no matter what your end goal may be. By taking care of your health, you set yourself up to work on goals and to thrive. In order to be successful with our health, we must plan for it. When we wing it, we usually aren't successful.

The key is to plan your wins in advance, and a big part of that is making your health your top priority. When you do that, you form your lifestyle around your wellness, and not surprisingly, your results take off. When you make this shift, you will see and feel the results right away!

Let me explain. Most people try to plug in their wellness (exercising, eating right, getting solid sleep, etc.) around their hectic schedules. But the problem is that, if we don't *plan* our wellness and, instead, try to wing it, we usually guarantee non-victory. We plan to "fit in our workout later," which usually leads to putting it off further, which then usually leads to "it's too late now, so I'll do it tomorrow." And then the same thing plays out the next day, until the days become weeks and then months and then years and then decades. And we find ourselves still over-weight and off our game.

Does this sound familiar? When we put our wellness and health at the center of our being, we then position ourselves to win as we plug in our lifestyle and career around our *wellness*.

WIN THE 2-PERSON RACE

Each day, most of us have a conscious, or subconscious, debate about whether we have time to exercise and to nurture ourselves. We need to get to work, get the kids ready for school, do laundry, clean the house, etc. So, our negative voice talks us out of making our wellness the top priority and, instead, keeps us operating with a focus on trying to fit wellness in around our lifestyle or career.

Here is one example of how the 2-Person Race can play out:

Version #1 of you skips your morning workout and leaves for the office at 7:30 a.m., because "today is going to be insanely busy, so I need to get to the office."

Version #2 of you knows it will be a crazy day at work but decides she needs to get energized and positive prior to heading into the office. She nails the morning workout and leaves for the office at 8:30 a.m.

But here is the interesting thing: In this example, if you take the time to nail your morning workout and nurture your energy and vibe, you will always catch up to the version of yourself who rushed into the day. How? Because your pace will be quicker, and your focus and productivity will be much better! No, I don't mean how fast you walk around your house or office. I mean your mental pace—your problem solving, the speed with which you plow through tasks, and your ability to pounce on opportunities.

The post-workout version of you will catch up to the non-workout version of you every day, and that will usually happen between noon and 2:00 p.m. You can then spend the final hours of your day crushing it and drastically outperforming the dragging version of you.

In addition, there is a bonus payoff! Instead of dragging into your evening, you'll still have energy left. How? By taking care of yourself, nailing your workouts, and dropping weight. This concept applies to any time you decide to work out. For some that may be midday, for others at night. The overall benefits are the same: increased energy, feeling good, and knowing that you are taking care of your health.

There is also a second bonus payoff! You receive a major lift in self-worth for doing your workout. You won't carry around any guilt, and you don't have to hear your negative voice playing the same old disempowering song of "you always say you're going to exercise, but you never do it." No shame, no guilt—just the pride of a job well done.

YOU HAVE PLENTY OF TIME: HARNESS THE POWER75

There are 168 hours per week, and we are all given a clean slate of these hours every week. People who are thriving (including hitting their goal weight, getting fit, and staying there) make the important decision to allocate a certain amount of time to exercise.

One of the non-truths our negative voice tells us is that we don't have time. Yes, we are all very busy, but, as I'm about to explain, we have around 75 hours per week of non-sleep and non-work time. The key question isn't "Do I have time?" The key question is "Am I guarding my time and using it to serve me versus steal from me?"

Let me explain what I mean by "The Power75." There are 168 hours per week (7 X 24). Most people sleep an average of seven hours per night, which is about 49 hours per week. 168 minus 49 equals roughly 120 hours (yes, I'm rounding up).

Most people work an average of nine hours per day, which is about 45 hours per week. (120 − 45 = 75.)

So, most of us have 75 hours per week (roughly 10.5 hours per day) of non-sleep and non-work time. I call these your Power75, or your 75 available hours to take your power back.

You have the power to use those 75 hours as you choose. One example of how to look at this is, if you do six 30-minute work-outs per week, that is only three out of your Power75 hours. It's a small investment in time, with huge payoffs as far as your energy, vibe, focus, longevity, and performance in all areas of life.

Some people may still think they do not have enough time within those Power75 hours. If this is your case, I invite you to look at how much time you are spending on activities that may not be as impactful on your health and ability to thrive (mainly watching TV or being on social media).

In order to get an idea of how much time you spend on non-sleep and non-work activities, please complete the following exercise:

Add up the hours you spend each week doing the following (be honest!):

1. Watching TV
2. Using the Internet (for entertainment)

The average American spends 4.5 hours per day watching TV or 31.5 hours per week! If you allocated just 30 minutes a day, six days each week, to exercise, you can see that it does not even take away that much time from watching TV! If you watch TV for 31.5 hours each week, even with adding in the time to exercise, you could still watch 28.5 hours of TV, but with the benefits of living a healthy lifestyle.

Even though our negative voice will try to convince us that we do not have enough time in the day, we really do! Harness this concept of the Power75, and you will be shocked at how much time you actually have and how impactful those hours can be.

EXPECT INITIAL PUSHBACK FROM FAMILY AND, POSSIBLY, YOUR BOSS

When you start making the shift from trying to fit your wellness in around your lifestyle and career to putting wellness in the middle, you will probably receive pushback. This is especially true for anyone who takes care of others in their household, like parents caring for children or children caring for their aging parents.

If your family has treated you as if you should be around seven days per week, 24 hours per day, then they will need to go through an adjustment period as you pull back. Yes, you will actually be unavailable for 30 minutes. And no, the world won't end. But once your home team or work team sees how energized and positive you are, they should not have a problem with you continuing to form your lifestyle and career around your wellness. Try this out for one week, and you will feel drastically better and be much more productive during the day.

Chapter Thirteen

KEY HABIT #9: COMMIT TO THE 7-DAY WEEK

World-class athletes and world-class *people* don't take days off from their wellness and self-care. That doesn't mean they are perfect, but they are fully committed, and they don't take days off. Why? Because days off hinder your ability to be your best and lead to wasted time and to living with regret.

By "no days off," I do not mean that you have to work out every day or that you cannot have days when you indulge in eating your favorite treat. It just means you don't take a day off from your health being a priority. You understand that your health is such a huge part of thriving that maintaining it becomes part of your daily life.

BE COMMITTED, NOT JUST INTERESTED

I love the following quote and suggest you read it several times:

"There's a difference between interest and commitment. When you're interested in doing something, you do it only when it's convenient. When you're committed to something, you accept no excuses, only results." — Author Unknown

When you're committed, you don't let your negative voice convince you that you don't have time to exercise, while you're also spending time watching TV or playing online each day. When you're committed, you'll follow my suggestions, like setting yourself up for success each night by preparing a water bottle, workout clothes, and healthy snacks for the next day, even though you're tired and just want to relax on the couch with a glass of wine. When you're committed, you're confident that you will achieve your goals, because you take 100% ownership of your results.

Most people who struggle with meeting their goals and thriving are living what I call four-, five- or six-day weeks. So, for four, five, or six days out of the week, they are focused on their healthy habits and their self-care. But then they take one, two, or three days off (usually the weekend) and cancel out all their results from their "on" days. Does this sound familiar?

The concept of committing to a 7-day week is simple, but don't let the simplicity fool you.

"The things that are easy to do are also easy not to do." — Jim Rohn

BE ONE VERSION OF YOURSELF

Part of the process of shifting to the 7-day week involves narrowing down to one version of yourself. Most people have two "versions" of themselves, and each one has a different approach to self-care. There is the version that prioritizes self-care, and there is the version that is lax on self-care. Typically, the version that prioritizes self-care is present mid-week, when you are able to follow a familiar schedule. The lax version presents itself on weekends, vacations, or even when traveling for work.

Most people are so lax with their health on the weekends that they end up canceling out all their hard work from during the week. It is almost as if you go up two steps during the week (results-wise) and then back down those two steps over the weekend. This leads to feeling less than amazing and to being a spectator of your best self. You deserve better, and the answer is to commit to one version of yourself.

Again, this does not mean you can never indulge or never fully rest! It means to find the balance that works for you! To attain an energy level of 5, to be your healthiest self, and to thrive, you deserve to narrow down to just one version of yourself: the fully committed-to-self-care version.

SET BARE MINIMUMS TO CREATE A SAFETY NET

Many people engage in all-or-nothing thinking when it comes to health. They are either fully committed or completely out, meaning that, if they miss one part of their plan, like skipping a workout or missing a day of work, they give up on the entire program. This all-or-nothing thinking leads to major fluctuations in weight, energy, and true happiness.

The way to beat this cycle and to help you commit to one version of yourself, committed seven days a week to your own well-being, is by identifying bare minimums. These are three to five health habits that you do no matter what (at the bare minimum). So, unless there is a huge emergency, you are doing them. This is how you can identify that balance with prioritizing your health. You are committed to doing these few things, and you know you can stick with them, even on weekends and on vacation.

Some examples of these bare minimum health habits are:

- Drinking eight glasses of water each day
- Getting seven hours of sleep each night
- Exercising 20 minutes, three days each week

Another form of a bare minimum is to follow what I call "The 5-Minute Rule." This is committing to do five minutes of your planned activity—no matter what.

Ninety percent of the battle with doing anything is just getting started. The 5-minute rule solves this common challenge. For example, when it comes to working out, on the days you're not feeling it and want to blow off your workout, just commit to moving for five minutes. Most of the time, once you start the workout, you begin to feel better, and, all of a sudden, five minutes leads to ten minutes, which leads to you doing your full workout. That can be a powerful personal-growth opportunity, because you feel great about yourself for fighting through your resistance and coming out the other side.

Find the bare minimums that will work for you. By committing to bare minimums, you guarantee that you are always committed to your health. This combination of committing to a 7-day week and leveraging the power of bare minimums will be rocket fuel for consistency and results on your journey to thrive.

Chapter Fourteen

KEY HABIT #10: PLAN FOR SUCCESS

The more you plan, the less you have to think, and the more you will stay on track.

Winging it in any area of our lives rarely leads to success. Without planning in advance, you are more or less guaranteeing non-victory and inadvertently guaranteeing a mediocre life. That is blunt, but true, and is why this chapter on planning is key to your ability to thrive.

"If you fail to plan, you are planning to fail." — Benjamin Franklin

PLANNING PRECEDES SUCCESS

Planning is pivotal to your consistency and is important, as far as implementing Key Habit #8 (forming your lifestyle and career around your wellness). When you make a plan about when you will exercise, what foods you will eat, what time you will wake up and go to sleep, and what actions you will take toward your specified goals, you are increasing the chances that you will actually do the work. Your plan adds structure to your mental game, allowing you to focus more on action and less on making decisions.

PLANNING = FREEDOM

Many people resist planning because they think it robs them of their freedom. They don't like being held back from exploring and going with the flow. But the irony is that, the more you plan, the more freedom you create. You remove the thought time and associated stress of decision-making, plus planning leads to more consistency in your self-care. That consistency leads to you performing mentally, physically, spiritually, and emotionally at your best, and with that, you increase your effectiveness and productivity (which creates more time and freedom in your schedule). It's a beautiful cycle of planning creating more and more freedom!

USE THE WIN TOMORROW CHECKLIST TO PLAN AND THRIVE

As I have mentioned, one of the keys to thriving is living a healthy lifestyle (exercising and eating well). The "Win Tomorrow Checklist" is a tool that helps you prepare for the next day, to increase your chances of success at prioritizing your health. It reminds you to get everything you will need to exercise ready, to make plans for what you will eat, and to plan what time you will go to sleep.

The reason this checklist works is that having everything on the list set up the night before leaves you in a great spot to avoid excuses, like "I can't find my sneakers," "I forgot to pack my lunch, so I will get take-out," etc. Avoiding those excuses means you have a better shot at "winning tomorrow!"

The key to staying consistent with the Win Tomorrow Checklist is to complete it at a set time each night (for example, right after finishing dinner). It takes about five or six minutes per day to complete and it sets you up for success.

Win Tommorrow Checklist							
	Completed? If so, check the box.						
Action Item:	Monday	Tuesday	Wednesday	Thursday	Friday	Saturday	Sunday
Get your water bottles ready.							
Get your healthy snacks ready.							
Make or plan your lunch.							
Get your workout clothes and sneakers ready.							
Schedule tomorrow's workout in your calendar.							
Set an exact bedtime for tonight.							

Access the Win Tomorrow Checklist online by going to:

www.12KeyHabits.com/Book

BOOKENDING YOUR DAY FOR SUCCESS

Another simple, but powerful, way to leverage planning as a way to crank up your results is to bookend your day for success. This means taking the time at key transitions in your day (morning, end of workday, and nighttime) to refocus to make sure you are on track to work toward meeting your goals.

The concept is simple, but don't let the simplicity fool you. Please keep this powerful quote from Jim Rohn (that I shared earlier) on your mind as you read this section:

"The things that are easy to do are also easy not to do." — Jim Rohn

A great way to do this is to create a one-page document and give it the title of "Bookending Your Day for Success." It will have three sections:

- Your Morning Routine
- Your End-of-Workday Routine
- Your Nighttime Routine

You should list 3–6 habits for both the Morning Routine and Nighttime Routine. You should also list the exact time you plan on doing each habit. You should list 2–4 habits for your End of Workday Routine, and also include the exact time you plan on doing each habit.

By writing or typing out your exact habits, you are creating three bookends around your day to maximize your follow-through, consistency, and success.

It's important that I point something out: If your negative voice is complaining that "this sounds hard," then here is my response: "Success is expensive, and it's not handed out—it's earned!" I don't mean expensive as far as your hard-earned money. I mean expensive as far as investing time, energy, focus, and follow-through. You are worth it, so tell your negative voice to take a hike and keep on reading.

Before you begin writing down your own habits for your document, I want to suggest one habit that will help you begin your day on a positive note.

First, I want to give you a heads up, so that you aren't shocked. Your negative voice may complain as I suggest this new change in habit, so here goes: Stop hitting the snooze button.

Hitting the snooze button is the first move in decreasing your self-worth, before you even get out of bed. You deserve better. Simply set the alarm and get out of bed.

If you want to achieve your goals, be the healthiest you can be, and thrive, then you have to do some challenging things as you elevate your game. One of them is to ditch the snooze habit.

Here is a simple tip: Put your alarm clock across the room, so you have to get out of bed to turn it off. This is simple, but it works.

EXAMPLE OF A BOOKENDING YOUR DAY FOR SUCCESS DOCUMENT

Morning Routine:

6:00 a.m. Wake up (no snooze)

6:15 a.m. Read my Declaration to Thrive (see after Conclusion)

6:25 a.m. Exercise

7:00 a.m. Shower

7:45 a.m. Breakfast

8:30 a.m. Launch my workday

End of Workday Routine:

5:00 p.m. Watch a 5-minute motivational video (see Chapter 19 for suggestions)

5:05 p.m. Read my Declaration to Thrive

5:15 p.m. Say to myself "Okay, work is over. It's time to shift into my personal life."

Nighttime Routine:

9:00 p.m. Shut off my phone for the night and have my last sip of water.

9:00 p.m. – 9:45 p.m. Watch a show or do something to relax

9:45 p.m. Get ready for bed

9:55 p.m. Read my Declaration to Thrive

10:00 p.m. Read positive content (no electronics) in bed

10:30 p.m. Fall asleep so that I get 7+ hours of sleep

It is not a coincidence that people who are thriving in life have planned out how to win. They detail it, and then they work the plan. Their success comes from their commitment to their plan.

SIMPLICITY WINS

The actions that you are planning to win tomorrow and to bookend your day for success with are not complicated tasks. We all get up at some point during the day and we all eat. In fact, these actions are often perceived as so simple that people don't make plans and just wing it. But in order to thrive, you need to be more purposeful about the flow of your day.

The more you plan, the fewer decisions you need to make. This simplifies your life, decreases your stress, and helps you avoid decision fatigue. It also sets you up to thrive.

ACCEPT THE 7-DAY PLANNING CHALLENGE

Take action by using the Win Tomorrow Checklist yourself. For the next seven days, commit to setting yourself up each evening for success with your health.

If the entire checklist seems overwhelming to you, break it down and start with 1–2 steps and then add on as you gain momentum. For example, start with getting your water bottles ready and commit to that for one week. Then the next week, you can add in getting your healthy snacks ready.

Follow through with this, and I think you will be hooked. Will it be easy? No. But remember that nothing worthwhile is easy. You are setting yourself up to nail a key part of thriving—living a healthy lifestyle. The more you work on your planning muscles, the easier it will be, so go for it!

Chapter Fifteen

KEY HABIT #11: SET INSANELY BIG GOALS

"Unless you try to do something beyond what you have already mastered, you will never grow." — Ronald Osborn

I read the words "Destined for Greatness" on a blanket that my wife, Karen, pulled out for our youngest son one morning when he was a baby. I loved seeing it. It made me think about the fact that, when we're young, we're told we can do anything we set our minds to. We're given the impression that we are "destined for greatness."

While this is actually true—we *do* all have the potential to achieve greatness—somewhere along the way, we pull back on shooting for the moon and, instead, just go with the flow. This is why creating "Insanely Big Goals" can help to re-spark that feeling of being destined for greatness.

Insanely Big Goals are goals that are so lofty that they make you uncomfortable. You want to reach them, but you know it will take hard work to get there. I believe that when we practice setting these Insanely Big Goals, they will become part of us and help us to continue to grow and achieve more, whatever that may be. This is what it means to thrive. People who push themselves to grow and develop are thriving.

FOUR WORDS THAT CHANGED MY LIFE: "YOU SHOULD DO IT!"

It was 1995, and I was sitting on the train in Boston, heading home from my finance job (I was a financial analyst at Fidelity Investments). A guy who had just run the Boston Marathon got on the train and sat right next to me. He was all sweaty, and his energy (given that he had just run a marathon) was amazing and very contagious.

I asked in amazement, "Did you just run the marathon?"

He said, "Yes, and it was the most amazing thing I've ever done!" He proceeded to tell me about his magical experience.

At the end of our conversation, he said to me, "You should do it!" It was a powerful moment that literally transformed my life.

I weighed 224 pounds (44 pounds more than I do today), and as you can imagine, was not exactly marathon-ready. I had played soccer in college and was fit (I had actually been an Academic All-American), but long work hours and poor nutrition had packed on the pounds. But I was so excited after seeing the look in this guy's eyes that I decided to set the Insanely Big Goal to run the Boston Marathon the following year. I actually called my dad that night to tell him the big news, and he was excited for me. That guy truly changed my life forever!

I ran my first Boston Marathon that next year (in 1996), and have now run every year since. I'm up to 27 straight Boston Marathons at the time of the publishing of this book in 2022. More important, I've run 26 straight years to raise funds for the Dana-Farber Cancer Institute, where my mom was treated for lung cancer when I was young. This was a big motivator for me personally, and it illustrates the power of finding your why. I have now kept 40 pounds off for over 27 years!

The simple statement "you should do it" transformed my life.

I'm not telling you this story in an effort to turn you into a marathon runner, or a runner at all. But I am telling you, "You should do it!" What is "it?" You decide, but set an Insanely Big Goal (one that really scares you and instigates action) and then go for it.

Maybe your Insanely Big Goal is walking continuously for ten minutes. Maybe it is walking a mile. Maybe your Insanely Big Goal is walking or running a 5K, a 10K, a half marathon, or a full marathon. Maybe it is to drink 8 glasses of water each day. Maybe your Insanely Big Goal is to eat vegetables three times each day. Maybe your Insanely Big Goal is to become the leader of a division of your company. Maybe your Insanely Big Goal is to start painting or learn how to play the piano.

As long as your Insanely Big Goal is a challenge, and is something you can measure (you can tell when it is accomplished), it is a great goal for you. The key is to set a firm goal and then get after it! This one decision to go after your goal could change your life, like the guy on the train in Boston in 1995 changed mine, by saying, "You should do it!"

"What would you attempt to do if you knew you could not fail?" — Unknown

I have Insanely Big Goals and am not afraid to share them with others. In fact, they are included in my Declaration to Thrive, which can be found after the Conclusion.

As you can read there, one of my Insanely Big Goals is to run 50 straight Boston Marathons for Dana-Farber Cancer Institute.

When I first started telling people that I wanted to run 50 straight Boston Marathons, they thought I had lost my mind. But I just went to work on the goal—one workout, one run, one day, etc., at a time. Then I hit five straight Boston Marathons, then 10 straight, then 15, then 20, and now, as of early 2022, I've completed 27 straight. I've already accomplished 54% of the initial Insanely Big Goal of running 50 straight Boston Marathons.

It's okay to be misunderstood when it comes to going after your goals. In fact, if you are not misunderstood by at least *some* people, you may be aiming too low.

So, even though people thought (and even still think) that my goal is an impossible one, I keep working toward it one small step at a time. By looking at it as a bunch of small wins and breaking it down into small steps, it makes the Insanely Big Goal seem more manageable.

TURN FEAR INTO YOUR SECRET WEAPON

Fear of failure robs many people of their ability to thrive. Their negative voices convince them that it's less risky to keep doing what they're doing than to risk the humiliation of not being successful in their efforts to go after their goals. This is a complete non-truth!

First, the only true failure is giving up after a setback. More than likely, you'll experience times when you are not progressing as you would like, or even times when you slip back into unhealthy patterns and habits. Remember that you are human and this is a natural part of any journey toward thriving. As long as you keep moving forward, you're learning. With enough persistence and the right tools (especially the mental ones you are learning in this book), success will be yours.

Second, the people who would judge you if you were to "fail" are not people you want to surround yourself with anyway. Why waste your time worrying about being judged? Your fans (people who truly care about you) won't judge you.

Third, most of our fears never come true anyway. We spend a great deal of time worrying about whether something is going to happen or not, and 90% of the time, none of it materializes.

Finally, you've never attempted to reach your goals by giving your positive voice control of the podium and combining that with the other habits to thrive. So, although your negative voice will feed you lines like "Haven't you tried this before and quit?", the truthful answer is *no*. You haven't tried *this* approach before, because *this* approach is completely different and sustainable. It's time to turn fear into your secret weapon!

The word "potential" is defined in *Webster's Dictionary* as "existing in possibility; capable of development into actuality." Here's something very exciting: we're all only using a small portion of our true potential!

I'm not saying this to freak you out or give your negative voice more material to lecture you about. I'm saying this because it's a *good* thing, that should get you excited about the future. I suggest, from this moment forward, that you shift from fearing failure to fearing not reaching your potential.

Just reading this should make you a bit uncomfortable, because most people want nothing to do with talking about reaching their potential. But what if, instead of running from the concept of reaching your potential, you ran toward it? What if, each day, you thought about how you could take actions that lead you closer and closer to your true potential? Your negative voice will try to convince you that it can't be this simple and that your time is better spent dwelling on the past. But, at this point, you know that's the road to nowhere.

Here's the fun part: the less of your potential you've reached so far, the more fired up you should be about your future, because of the tremendous progress you are going to make!

There is no greater regret later in life than not having lived up to your potential. Take the time now to change the outcome and see what the future will bring. This should get you excited to take action! If you'll give yourself the gift of converting your fear of failure into a fear of not living up to your potential, then you'll have discovered a secret weapon in your pursuit of becoming who you deserve to be!

How about you? What huge goals have you made in the past that your negative voice talked you out of? If your negative voice has been telling you that it's too late or that you don't know how to make Insanely Big Goals or that you couldn't possibly achieve them, you need to put your positive voice at the podium and just get started.

GOAL-SETTING AND GOAL-ACHIEVING

A great way to identify your Insanely Big Goal is to ask, "What, why, when, and how?"

- **What** is the goal?
- **Why** do you want to achieve the goal?
- **When** do you plan on achieving the goal?
- **How** do you plan on achieving the goal (tools, strategies, and habits)?

Here are seven key areas of your life that you can identify goals for: health, family, career, relationships, financial, growth (personal and professional), and joy and happiness. You don't have to have goals for all seven areas. Maybe start with two, three or four.

Once you have made a list of goals, choose one Insanely Big Goal, and write it down. Goals that are not written down are still dreams. You have to write them out, or type them out, in order to set them in motion to be actualized. Having no written goals, or having weak goals, leads to unorganized effort, which leads to weak results. But Insanely Big Goals that make you uncomfortable and stretch you, command more focus, attention, and follow-through, and lead to exponentially better results.

What big dreams do you have asleep inside of you? Every one of us had big dreams at some point. Every one of us has the strength inside to accomplish anything we set our minds to. You were destined for greatness when you were born, and I know today is the day to begin dreaming big again and to take the first step toward making those dreams happen. Yes, you can!

> "The greatest danger for most of us is not that our aim is too high and we miss it. Rather, it's that we aim too low and we reach it." — Michelangelo

Chapter Sixteen

KEY HABIT #12: USE POSITIVE CONTENT TO WIN THE MENTAL GAME

At this point, you realize the importance of winning the mental game in order to thrive. A key part of winning the mental game is using external resources (books, videos, coaches, friends, etc.) to enhance your positivity and mindset. Most positive and high-energy people (me included) use positive content as rocket fuel to keep themselves feeling energized and on fire.

BECOME A POSITIVE CONTENT MACHINE

"Stand guard at the gates to your mind!" — Jim Rohn

Pay attention to what you're watching, what you're listening to, and what you're reading, for additional opportunities to crank up your positivity, energy, mood, weight loss, fitness, health, and life! Make a list of what you watch, listen to, and read and then mark them with a P for positive or an N for negative. This will help you visualize how much positive and negative content you are exposed to. Each time we consume content, we are either lifting ourselves up or dragging ourselves down. So the more positive content you consume, the more you will be lifted up!

"Turn your car into a mobile classroom." — Zig Ziglar

Your ability to thrive will take off when you swap many of your negative sources of content for positive ones. A great way to absolutely nail this key habit, is to schedule 10–30 minutes of positive content per day in your calendar.

If your negative voice just scoffed at that, then, as you have done before, add up the amount of time you spend watching TV or on social media each day, and you will see that you can fit this time in if thriving is a top priority. You can listen to positive content while going for a walk, while cleaning your house, or while cooking dinner. You can read positive content on a break from work. You can choose more positive content to watch when you watch television. You can listen to positive content in your car or on a bus or train. This habit will leave you in a much better mood each day, and when you layer this habit on top of your daily workout and other healthy habits, you will become the most positive person in the room.

FIND AND FOLLOW POSITIVE CONTENT GUIDES

Finding positive content can be fun! There is so much out there, so look and see what speaks to you.

It helps to find "positive content guides." These are people who are always learning and growing and who provide a daily or weekly email or video, and only share valuable and powerful content on their social media page.

Here are a few suggestions for free daily emails:

1. Me (subscribe to my Daily Coaching Video): https:// www.12KeyHabits.com/DailyCoaching/
2. Darren Hardy (subscribe to Darren Daily): https://go. darrenhardy.com/darrendaily/
3. John Maxwell (subscribe to Minute with Maxwell): https://johnmaxwellteam.com/minute/

Go to www.12KeyHabits.com/PCGuides to access my updated list of new and positive newsletters to add to your day.

Give this habit a try for one week and see what this does for your energy and mood, along with your overall goals to thrive! Remember, garbage in equals garbage out, and positivity in equals positivity out!

CONCLUSION

I wrote this book because I truly believe that everyone has it in them to thrive! You don't need to be perfect as you work toward improving and taking action on the 12 Key Habits to Thrive. In fact, your challenges along the way just mean you are human. We all stumble, but what really matters is that we keep pushing forward and do the best we can.

And that will look different on different days. Some days you will succeed at all twelve of the 12 Key Habits to Thrive, and some days you will only be able to take action on one or two. Your pace doesn't matter—all that matters is that there is forward progress. Slow and steady truly does win the race.

I am honored and blessed to have guided you through this book because I have traveled the same journey. I get it. I understand what it feels like to re-start and to be what appears to be a far distance from thriving. But I have also used these 12 Key Habits to Thrive myself to transform personally and professionally, and I have sustained them for over 25 years. You deserve to be next!

You are now ready to reveal your best self and thrive! Your lack of thriving up through this point was not a product of anything being wrong with you. You don't lack willpower or drive, and you are certainly not lazy. Those are all non-truths from your negative voice. You never needed to change; you simply deserved to reveal who you already are (powerful, smart, athletic, healthy, driven, kind, etc.). All you lacked prior to reading this book were the tools (mostly mental tools) to thrive.

You now have these tools and can be 100% in control of your energy, vibe, health, happiness, and future! Is that scary? Absolutely! But as I mentioned earlier in the book, when was the last time you did something great in your life without being scared? Being scared is a sign that you are on the cusp of a major breakthrough, so embrace it.

Remember these key concepts and tools you have just learned:

1. You have the power to re-start anytime. You can write a new story, become the best version of yourself, and thrive, and you can start today!

2. The most important decision of your life happens every day: your Voice Choice. Always strive to choose your positive voice over your negative voice.

3. Actions are important when it comes to thriving, but there are two key steps prior to taking action: choosing your voice and choosing your thoughts. Your voice

choice dictates your thoughts, and your thoughts dictate your actions, so you want to make sure your positive voice is at the podium of your mind so that your thoughts and actions are coming from a place of positivity.

4. You don't need to change (there was never anything wrong with you). You simply deserve to reveal who you already are. Treat yourself as if you already are who you have the potential to be! You really are already that person—you just need to peel off the layers to reveal her or him.

True happiness and contentment aren't achieved through reaching a destination or specific outcome. Your happiness is a product of your voice choice and thought choice, and you are 100% in control of both. I proudly send you off on your journey to thrive by re-sharing a powerful quote from earlier in the book:

"It's never too late to be who you might have been." – George Eliot

So hit the re-start button, nail your voice choice, focus on your energy, control your stress, have an attitude of gratitude, upgrade your team and embrace being a leader, embrace being your own effort-based head coach, exercise and be a random acts of fitness machine, form your lifestyle/career around your wellness, commit to the 7-day week, plan for success, set insanely big goals, and use positive content to win the mental game.

Now is truly your time to thrive!

MY DECLARATION TO THRIVE

You may have noticed that one of the actions in my bookending my day for success plan is to read my "Declaration to Thrive" three times each day. This declaration is a two-page document that defines my intention to thrive. It includes the things that motivate me (my inspiration for wanting to thrive, my favorite quotes, my mantras, etc.) It is an evolving document that I add to as I find new content that inspires me.

I read my declaration three times daily as part of my Morning Routine, End-of-Workday Routine, and Nighttime Routine.

Remember, there is not really a right way to create your Declaration to Thrive—just the right way for you. Your declaration will ideally have your "why" (I have a picture of my wife, Karen, and our three kids at the top of mine). It will also have your mantra (if you have one), your favorite quotes, rules to live by (you can call each section whatever you want), your goals, and anything else that gets you motivated and inspired.

Again, this is an evolving document, so don't let your negative voice make you feel overwhelmed or try to compare your first document to mine. Your first draft may include a picture of what is most important to you plus three quotes. That is great! You are out of the gate, and you can keep evolving it from there. My version, which you are about to read, is probably the twentieth version of my declaration and incorporates decades of researching and practicing ways to thrive.

Here it is:

MY TOP 3 PRIORITIES (PERSONALLY & PROFESSIONALLY):

1. To be the absolute best version of myself (mentally, physically, spiritually & emotionally)!
2. Personally: To support Karen, Alex, Ben, and Adeline in being the absolute best versions of themselves! Professionally: To support my team in being the absolute best versions of themselves!
3. To positively impact as many people as humanly possible!

12 RULES TO THRIVE

1. Nail my voice choice (choose my positive voice over my negative voice)!
2. Have fun!

3. Try my best!
4. Treat everyone (including myself) with respect!
5. Treat everyone (including myself) as if they already are who they have the potential to be!
6. Leave everyone (and everything) better than I found them!
7. How much I care about others and uniquely see them and understand them (empathy) will dictate how many people allow me to serve them and positively impact them (and their family)!
8. Extreme gratitude is key to true happiness! Don't ever forget opening up the fridge and seeing just ketchup and butter—you are now Blessed Beyond Comprehension (BBC)!
9. Always keep your energy bucket full because you can't give away what you don't have!
10. Live like a professional athlete by perpetually nurturing your mind and body!
11. Earn your healthy longevity! You don't feel your age—you feel your habits!
12. Out-care, out-serve, out-give, our-prepare, out-coach, and out-lead everyone else!

MY INSANELY BIG GOALS:

1. Be one of the most energetic, healthy, optimistic, happy, and inspiring people in the world!
2. Positively impact 100 million lives by 2030 through Breakthrough Health's patented software system

MY DECLARATION TO THRIVE

(EnergyUP.co, BeatDiabetes.com, BeatDepression.com, etc.)!

3. Sell 100 million "12 Key Habits" books by 2033 (not to sell books, but to use books as vehicles to reach and positively impact lives)!

4. Run 50 straight Boston Marathons for Dana-Farber Cancer Institute (in memory of my mom)! So, I will run my last one when I'm 73—in 2045.

5. Positively impact 1 billion people by the end of my life (at approx. age 100—so by 2072)!

8 KEY STEPS TO THRIVE (THEY FLOW IN ORDER):

1) Voice Choice 2) Thoughts 3) Actions 4) Results 5) Self-Worth 6) Self-Belief 7) Leadership 8) Positive Impact

"To give anything less than your best is to sacrifice the gift." — Steve Prefontaine

"What would you attempt to do if you knew you could not fail?" — Unknown

"Only those who will risk going too far can possibly find out how far one can go." — T.S. Eliot

"The gull sees farthest who flies highest." — Richard Bach

"Everyone gets the good stuff! Treat the garbage man the same way you treat a CEO. Giving respect is free and easy!" — Don Roche

"If you have your health, someone to love, a roof over your head and food in the fridge, then you have everything you need for an amazing life. Don't ever forget that!" — Dory Roche

"You can be anything you want to be if you believe in yourself, treat people right, work really hard and always do the right thing." — Dory Roche

"Unless you try to do something beyond what you have already mastered, you will never grow." — Ronald Osborn

"Your future is created by what you do today, not tomorrow." — Robert Kiyosaki

"If you want to be happy, set a goal that commands your thoughts, liberates your energy and inspires your hopes" — Andrew Carnegie

"Stand guard at the gates to your mind!" — Jim Rohn

"Your energy announces you to the room before you speak." — Unknown

"To achieve what 1% of the population achieves, you must do what 99% of the population is not willing to do."

"You miss 100% of the shots you don't take." — Wayne Gretzky

"You only live once, but if you do it right, once is enough." — Mae West

"It's not the critic who counts; not the man who points out how the strong man stumbles, or where the doer of deeds could have done them better. The credit belongs to the man who is actually in the arena, whose face is marred by dust and sweat and blood; who strives valiantly; who errs, who comes short again and again, because there is no effort without error and shortcoming; but who does actually strive to do the deeds; who knows great enthusiasms, the great devotions; who spends himself in a worthy cause; who at the best knows in the end the triumph of high achievement, and who at the worst, if he fails, at least fails while daring greatly, so that his place shall never be with those cold and timid souls who neither know victory nor defeat." — Theodore Roosevelt

"Twenty years from now you will be more disappointed by the things that you didn't do than by the ones you did do. So throw off the bowlines. Sail away from the safe harbor. Catch the trade winds in your sails. Explore. Dream. Discover." — Mark Twain

MANTRAS:

Use Your Gift! • Earn Your Awesome! • Be the Most Positive Person in the Room!

5 KEY DAILY ACTIONS THAT MAKE SUCCESS INEVITABLE:

1. I focus only on my controllables: my voice choice, attitude, habits, and effort!
2. I jump into each day with positive energy, extreme gratitude, and relentless optimism!
3. I work hard and I ignore the doubters as I chase down my Insanely Big Goals!
4. I focus on closing my potential gap and making a positive impact!
5. I embrace being a leader, and I pay the fees every day to be a World-Class Guide!

"This is the beginning of a new day. You have been given this day to use as you will. You can waste it or use it for good. What you do today is important because you are exchanging a day of your life for it. When tomorrow comes, this day will be gone forever; in its place is something that you have left behind...let it be something good." — Heartsill Wilson

Note: Above is the end of my Declaration to Thrive. To access my updated Declaration to Thrive go to www.12KeyHabits.com/Declaration

BONUS HABITS

I have covered the 12 Key Habits to Thrive in the main content of this book. These habits are at the core of what you need to incorporate into your life in order to meet your goals and to thrive. The bonus habits, that I have provided below, are additional tools and ideas that you can use to help you focus on your goals. Choose the ones that apply to you and use them! These are things that you can revisit and apply as needed on your journey to thrive.

BONUS HABIT #1: LIVE LIKE A PROFESSIONAL ATHLETE

It's time to think, act, live, and be like a professional athlete!

Pretend that you just woke up from being in a coma for two months. Your family and friends are overwhelmed with joy to see you are awake. Although you have a long road back to being fully recovered, you are now ready to start and get back to 100% health.

Now I want you to think of your favorite sport. Let's say it's swimming.

A few days after waking up from your coma, your family and close friends start asking you, "When do you think you can get back in the pool?" They then explain that you are a professional swimmer and that you're the most decorated Olympic athlete in history. You are Michael Phelps, and you have won 23 gold medals.

Your negative voice may think this is ridiculous, but your negative voice is the reason you have struggled with reaching your goals, so try to keep an open mind.

If you woke up from being in a coma and were told, and then believed, that you were a professional athlete, then, from that point on, you would focus on your health and nurturing your body and your mind. This is how strong your mind can be! You would believe that performing at your best is what you love to do, and you would act like a professional athlete. To thrive in the pool, you have to be all in—on your sleep, your hydration, your nutrition, your exercise, and most importantly, your mindset.

Now, consider the fact that, whatever your job is (corporate, teacher, nurse, mom, etc.), your ability to perform at your best is also tied to your body and your mind.

You can, and deserve to, harness the professional athlete mindset as you use the 12 Key Habits to Thrive to reinvent yourself, drop weight for good, and reach your goals. From today on, you are a professional athlete, who nurtures your body and your mind! I am not talking about perfectionism. I am simply talking about making nurturing your body and your mind your top priority.

One way to help you live like a professional athlete is to focus on viewing your time and energy in three phases:

1. Preparation (practice time)
2. Rest and rejuvenation (recharge time)

3. Game time (the key part of your day, when you need
    to be at your best)

Preparation is when you are using self-care habits (water, sleep, healthy nutrients, exercise, etc.) and positive content for personal and professional development (books, articles, videos, seminars, etc.) to improve your skills, abilities, attitude, and, most importantly, your mindset.

Rest and rejuvenation time is when you are recharging your battery through sleep, meditation, and not thinking about your job.

Game time is when you need to be at your best. These are the most important times of your day, when you need to have energy, positivity, optimism, and focus, in order to perform and serve at your best.

To close your potential gap (between who you are and who you have the potential to be), it's imperative that you realize what phase you are in and to focus your time and energy only on that phase. This one action alone will be a game changer!

One more important point: Applying this concept is not about only eating healthy and going to bed early. You can still enjoy yourself (in moderation) as you adopt the professional athlete approach to nurturing your body and mind. The main goal is to prioritize your health and well-being.

BONUS HABIT #2: NUTRITION IS IMPORTANT

DON'T USE EXERCISE AS AN EXCUSE TO EAT BADLY

You may recall a controversial article that was on the cover of *Time* in 2010 stating, "Why Exercise Won't Make You Thin!" That bold statement was more to sell magazines than to try to argue that exercise doesn't work for weight loss. The core of the article, however, was that many people use their exercise habits as their excuse to eat badly.

Is that you?

If you've been completing three interval workouts and three No Excuses Workouts (strength training) each week for at least two weeks, and you have not lost weight or inches, or cranked up your energy, then it is time to evaluate your nutrition.

You may be using exercise as a reason to eat badly or to increase your caloric intake.

I suggest you make a firm and serious commitment to yourself right now to put an end to it. Here's why: life's too short to spin your wheels. When you nail your workouts (like taking two steps up the stairs) and then counter that with bad nutrition (like taking two steps back down the stairs), your net fitness and weight loss results are zero.

I want you to take a few minutes right now to honestly ask yourself if you're using exercise as your excuse to eat badly. Being candid with, and accountable to, yourself will finally allow your rocket to leave the pad!

THE 5 TRIGGERS OF BAD NUTRITIONAL CHOICES

If you look back at the times so far this year that you have made bad nutritional choices, I'm sure that, 90% of the time, one or some of the following five things happened:

1. You didn't have breakfast within one hour of waking up.
2. You hadn't eaten every two to three hours that day.
3. You weren't well hydrated.
4. You hadn't slept at least seven hours the night before.
5. You hadn't exercised.

Eating badly isn't the product of some weird gene you have, nor is it due to lack of self-control. Most of the time, it's simply due to a lack of being aware of the circumstances (some that are not even directly tied to food) that lead you to making bad food choices.

If you want to be successful with ensuring you provide your body with good nutrition, you need to be mindful of how you are going through your day.

8 KEY NUTRITIONAL HABITS TO MAKE HEALTHY CHOICES AND THRIVE

There are eight habits that are key to having the strong mindset to turn food into rocket fuel. If you are not in a mentally strong place, then it's nearly impossible to win the nutrition battle. That is why I want you to focus on these eight key nutritional habits to achieve the mindset needed to use food as nutrients to thrive.

I have listed these in order of importance:

1. Complete 5–6 workouts per week.
2. Sleep at least 7 hours per night.
3. Hydrate all day long.
4. Eat breakfast within one hour of waking up.
5. Eat every 2–3 hours throughout the day.
6. Limit yourself to one dessert per week (have a healthy snack on the other nights).
7. Control your portions.
8. Improve the quality of what you eat (more whole foods and fewer processed foods).

NUTRITION LOCK-IN SCORE

I created the Nutrition Lock-In Score to guide you in tracking the timing of what you put in your body, the quality of what you put in your body, and the portions you consume. Food is fuel, and it has the potential to increase your weight loss and energy, so use this tool as a guide to help with your nutrition.

Please don't let the simplicity of this tool and of the 8 Key Nutritional Habits fool you. They are both simple but highly effective!

Here is how it works (the score is for one week at a time):

- You get 1 point if the meal is healthy, and you have a healthy portion.
- The max score is 35, because you can earn points for 7 breakfasts, 7 lunches and 7 dinners per week (21 potential points) and for your daily mid-morning and mid-afternoon snacks (14 potential points).
- Desserts: If you had more than one dessert in the week, subtract 1 point for each additional dessert beyond the one weekly dessert.

Here is an example: All of your major meals were healthy but one (accumulating 20 points) and all of your snacks were healthy but one (13 points), for a total of 33. But you had 3 desserts, so you subtract 1 point per extra dessert, so your final score is 31.

Your score tells you how committed you are to your nutrition.

- Not Committed: Your score is less than 30.
- Committed: Your score is between 30 and 33.
- Fully Committed: Your score is 34 or 35.

Focus on getting your score to 34 or 35, and you will be shocked at how great you feel and how much that positively impacts your weight loss, fitness, energy, and health!

CALL TO ACTION: ACCEPT THE 70-DAY THRIVE CHALLENGE

At this point, you have all the tools and strategies you need to reveal your best self, hit your goal weight, crank up your energy, feel remarkable, and truly thrive!

With that, I invite you to participate in a 70-Day Thrive Challenge. This is ten weeks of you fully committing to the 12 Key Habits (not being perfect—just fully committing) so that you can shock yourself with your results and how much better you feel.

Please go to www.PeakLockIN.com/70DayChallenge

to join the next challenge.

Let's do this!

ADDITIONAL PROGRAMS

Live Events (Retreats, Thrive Academy, etc.) at Jonathan's special property in Vermont:

www.PeakLockIN.com/ and click on "Live Events in Vermont"

Jonathan's 1-on-1 Peak Performance Coaching and Team Coaching:

www.PeakLockIN.com/Coaching

Have Jonathan do a Keynote Speaking Engagement at your company or event:

www.PeakLockIN.com/Keynotespeaking

Made in the USA
Middletown, DE
04 March 2024

50222856R00089